P5 eHealth: An Agenda for the Health Technologies of the Future

Gabriella Pravettoni • Stefano Triberti
Editors

P5 eHealth: An Agenda for the Health Technologies of the Future

Springer Open

Editors
Gabriella Pravettoni
Department of Oncology and
Hemato-Oncology
University of Milan
Milan, Italy

Applied Research Division for Cognitive
and Psychological Science
European Institute of Oncology (IEO)
IRCCS
Milan, Italy

Stefano Triberti
Department of Oncology and
Hemato-Oncology
University of Milan
Milan, Italy

Applied Research Division for Cognitive
and Psychological Science
European Institute of Oncology (IEO)
IRCCS
Milan, Italy

ISBN 978-3-030-27993-6 ISBN 978-3-030-27994-3 (eBook)
https://doi.org/10.1007/978-3-030-27994-3

This Springer imprint is published by the registered company Springer Nature Switzerland AG.
The registered company address is: Gewerbestrasse 11, 6330 Cham, Switzerland

Preface

The idea of this book emerged within the discussion of the implementation and resources of a Europe-funded project (IManage), especially regarding the utilization of an eHealth platform. eHealth is regarded as a fundamental resource for care nowadays, to the point that a growing number of scientific publications involve some form of web-based and/or immersive technologies devoted to improve patient adherence to treatment and healthy activities, patient education, and even the monitoring of mental health outcomes such as stress, emotions, as well as biases potentially affecting health-related decision-making.

However, by analyzing the literature on these topics, we realized that eHealth evolution still tends mostly to the implementation and exploitation of technological advancement, but the consideration of behavioral, psychological, and emotional aspects often remains on the background. Some years ago, the first editor of this book proposed the concept of P5 medicine, by adding one-fifth requirement for the evolution of medicine to the original ones in the well-known P4 approach. This last P was related to *psycho-cognitive* characteristics of patients; specifically, besides being preventive, personalized, predictive, and participatory, medicine should become able to:

1. Engage patients in personalized treatment as well as management plans: patients should become competent, active, responsible managers of their own health
2. Analyze and improve quality of life not as a secondary but as a primary objective of the care process

In order to achieve such aims, medicine should turn to psychology and cognitive sciences in order to understand how patients interpret and use information on their own healthcare and also how they do develop intentions and behavior which could be more or less useful toward their health and wellness improvement. Also, healthcare should develop and master its own techniques and psychometric instruments to be included in care practices to account for these aspects.

Originally, the P5 approach as described here was not explicitly related to technology, but of course, eHealth constitutes an unprecedented opportunity to pursue all the five Ps within the healthcare process. In light of this concept, the present book is aimed to give examples, guidelines, suggestions, and methods to achieve the development of health technologies able not only to support health management but also to capture and exploit the personologic uniqueness of each individual.

In the contemporary scenario, where the main challenge faced by the healthcare systems worldwide is not to cure a specific disease but to support the management of incurable, chronic conditions and to guarantee long-term care to patients and survivors, such approach could be crucial to ensure that health technologies will be used and demonstrate their utility in the long term.

In this book, each one of the 5 Ps will be explained in depth by the authors with a specific expertise, with a focus on how they could be achieved through the use of specific health technologies; secondarily, other contributions will explore important aspects of eHealth design, implementation, and management.

Chapter 1, written by the editors of this book, will present the P5 approach and link it to eHealth, along with a short resume of health technologies themselves and considerations about their present and future.

Chapter 2 will present the IManage project and its technologies, in order to elaborate on them as an example of eHealth platform that has been designed and will be improved exactly on the basis of the P5 approach.

Chapter 3 will explore the first P, namely, *prevention*: the opportunities of new technologies for the forecast of future diseases and health issues will be described.

Chapter 4 will explore the concept of *personalized* medicine and will show that digital media can be used by patients both to express themselves and to communicate with health providers and by health providers to better comprehend patients' personal experience.

Chapter 5 will be focused on computational model and approaches to analyze and interpret data in order to *predict* future state of patients and illnesses; according to recent studies, this could be done not only with genetic and anatomical data but also with psychological and behavioral information.

Chapter 6 will present and comment on examples of specific technological features (coming from IManage technologies again and from other digital solutions) that could be used effectively to promote the active *participation* of patients to their own care, in order to advance toward activation and engagement.

Chapter 7 will explore the *psycho-cognitive* characteristics of patients, by remarking upon the importance of them in diagnosis and intervention; secondarily, persuasive technologies will be presented as one possible resource toward the implementation of behavioral and cognitive strategies within the technologies themselves, in order to promote positive behavioral change in patients.

Chapter 8 will present innovative technologies used in oncology and cancer care; indeed, also, diagnostic and research technologies should be taken into consideration when considering health technologies.

Chapter 9 will provide a brief history of the disciplines related to technology evaluation (e.g., ergonomics, usability, user experience), in order to promote the adoption of state-of-the-art methodologies for the design and evaluation of P5 eHealth solutions.

Chapter 10 will explore ethical issues related to the adoption of different health technologies (e.g., privacy) and suggest ways to effectively deal with them at an organizational level.

In the end, the objective of the present book is to set the grounds for the further development of P5 as a concept able to guide the growth of medicine, as well as the virtuous utilization of technological tools with the aim of improving human health and well-being.

Milan, Italy

Gabriella Pravettoni
Stefano Triberti

Contents

About the Editors

Gabriella Pravettoni, Ph.D. is Full Professor of Psychology of Decision-Making and Director of the Department of Oncology and Hemato-oncology (DIPO) at the University of Milan, Italy. She is also Director of the Applied Research Division for Cognitive and Psychological Science at the European Institute of Oncology (IEO) IRCCS and Coordinator of the doctorate course "FOLSATEC" (Foundations of the Life Sciences and Their Ethical Consequences) at SEMM (European School of Molecular Medicine), Milan, Italy. Her main research activities focus on medical humanities, in particular on patient empowerment and wellbeing, cognitive processes, decisions in medicine, errors prevention, and eHealth. She has authored more than 260 scientific publications to date on these topics.

Stefano Triberti holds a Ph.D. in Psychology. He is a Researcher at the Department of Oncology and Hemato-oncology of the University of Milan, Italy, and collaborates with the Applied Research Division for Cognitive and Psychological Science, European Institute of Oncology IRCCS, Milan, Italy. His research activities focus mainly on ergonomics and user experience of new technologies for medicine and healthcare (eHealth) and the usage of innovative resources to promote health and well-being. He has authored around 70 scientific publications on these topics.

About the Editors

Part I
Foundations for P5 eHealth

Chapter 1
A "P5" Approach to Healthcare and Health Technology

Gabriella Pravettoni and Stefano Triberti

1 Introduction

The main challenge faced by healthcare systems worldwide is not the cure of specific diseases but the management of chronic illness emerging from diseases that are treatable but incurable. This scenario requires the health providers to maintain long-term relationship with the patient, who has to learn how to manage symptoms, organize treatment adherence (e.g., taking medications regularly), and cope with stress and negative emotions as well.

The literature agrees that patients themselves should not be seen as passive recipients of care, but rather they should become "active" (Hibbard et al. 2007; Remmers et al. 2009), "empowered" (Anderson and Funnell 2010; Pravettoni 2016; Renzi et al. 2017), or "engaged" (Barello et al. 2012; Graffigna et al. 2016) in their own care in order to recover a positive approach to everyday life issues and to the management of illness and the treatment as well.

This theoretical approach to healthcare lays its own roots in the patient-centered approach to medicine. Patient-centered medicine emphasizes the limitations of a disease-centered approach to medicine, namely, the idea according to which health practitioners should focus their activity on the recognition and treatment of the symptoms only. On the contrary, patient-centered medicine attributes importance to the recognition and appreciation of patients' values, desires, expectations, personal objectives, and lived experience in general.

On this basis, patients deserve to be made active participants in the decisions related to their own care plan. Historically, patient-centered medicine emerged dur-

G. Pravettoni (✉) · S. Triberti
Department of Oncology and Hemato-Oncology, University of Milan, Milan, Italy

Applied Research Division for Cognitive and Psychological Science, European Institute of Oncology (IEO) IRCCS, Milan, Italy
e-mail: gabriella.pravettoni@ieo.it; stefano.triberti@unimi.it

G. Pravettoni, S. Triberti (eds.), *P5 eHealth: An Agenda for the Health Technologies of the Future*, https://doi.org/10.1007/978-3-030-27994-3_1

ing the second half of the 1900s (Balint et al. 1970); Levenstein (1984) elaborated some of the most important theoretical principles of the approach, namely, the belief that both physician's and patient's *agendas* should be recognized and integrated in medical care. Specifically, the patient's agenda could be described in terms of three main domains:

1. The cognitive sphere or the patient's ideas about his/her own condition and the "folk models" about health and illness.
2. The emotional sphere or patient's feeling, emotions, and affective reactions to illness and care.
3. The expectation sphere or patients' objectives and desires about the processes and the outcomes of care.

Today, patient-centered medicine is worldwide recognized as a fundamental component of the healthcare system or better as the correct, desirable, and more ethical approach to healthcare; however, there is still uncertainty around the actual meaning of "patient centeredness" for health practitioners, patients, and health organizations (Bardes 2012; Hanyok et al. 2012; Miller et al. 2015). According to Liberati and colleagues (Liberati et al. 2015), a review of patient-centered interventions highlights at least two main approaches, namely, the dyadic and the organizational ones.

The dyadic approach to patient-centered medicine includes those interventions focused on strengthening and empowering patient-doctor communication or in other words those interventions that focus on individual experience of illness, therapy administration, and treatment management, for example, basing on a "narrative medicine" approach (Fioretti et al. 2016). Dyadic studies are usually centered on clinical encounters and individual interactions/communications; they explore innovative ways of creating a positive alliance between the patient and the health provider, and they report outcomes showing how the interventions influence (or not) therapy effectiveness and well-being outcomes.

On the other hand, organizational interventions move the focus of inquiry from clinical encounters to the overall healthcare context; in other words, they intervene at the level of procedures, practices, policies, organizational boundaries, and roles and the communication of the medical offer in order to improve patient centeredness at the level of organizations and their services.

Both these approaches have specular strengths and limitations. Dyadic patient-centered approaches may fail to recognize organizational factors that influence patients' well-being and/or effectiveness of illness management independently of the quality of the communication with the health provider (e.g., complex time schedules in the care facility), and also they do not consider additional important figures (e.g., caregivers); on the other hand, organizational patient-centered approaches do not address how practitioners carry out care in their local context nor do they capture what patients perceive as actually significant along their care path.

On this basis, it appears evident that a mature approach to patient-centered medicine should encompass both dyadic and organizational aspects; probably, this could be done by adopting a different stance, not focused on the specific type of intervention but rather on general features healthcare interventions should have in order to promote patient centeredness. The P5 approach to medicine does exactly that and will guide the contributions featured in this book.

2 P5 Medicine

The approach to medicine that is taken as a main guideline for theory and practice in the present book lies its roots in the evolution of medicine as a scientific activity. Professor Leeroy Hood, a pioneer in systems biology, theorized that modern medicine was evolving from P0 to P4 medicine (Hood and Galas 2008; Hood 2009, 2013); from a biological point of view, P0 medicine or the traditional approach was focused on individual analysis of "one cell or one protein," while the availability of technology-conveyed data around diseases and patients allows researchers and health providers to adopt a systems, holistic approach to diagnosis and treatment. Hood thought that future medicine would become more and more predictive, personalized, preventive, and participatory. Already in Hood's writings, but also in subsequent studies on the topic, these concepts transcended systems biology to embrace multiple disciplines and approaches involved in promoting healthcare (Cesario et al. 2014; Pulciani et al. 2017).

The **preventive** (cfr. Chap. 3) property of medicine refers to its ability to proactively (not only reactively) address diseases. According to Hood, by knowing the molecular picture of the patient and by using a systemic approach to its condition, it is possible to anticipate diseases as well as relapses or other modifications to overall health status. In the P5 approach, such characteristic extends to environmental, social, and psychological aspects of patients' experience; indeed, not only biological events can be anticipated but also changes in environment or psychological status (e.g., onset of depression, emotional reactions to the diagnosis, etc.), so to project therapy interventions that address pathology and issues before they actually manifest themselves.

Personalized medicine (cfr. Chap. 4) was originally proposed in the field of genetics, in the sense that by the application of nanogenomics and nanoproteomics, it is possible to tailor medical interventions to the specific molecular picture of the individual (Eisen et al. 1998; Nicolini et al. 2012); also this concept has evolved toward a consideration of the patient as a whole, so that "tailoring interventions" on people means designing them by taking into considerations patients' abilities, contexts, needs, and decision-making priorities (Cutica et al. 2014; Renzi et al. 2016).

Medicine should become more and more **predictive** (cfr. Chap. 5) which means it will employ the information arising from genome sequences and longitudinal molecular, cellular, and phenotypic measurements to provide baseline values that can be defined as health/wellness and then used to identify subsequent transitions to disease. Consistently with its original formulation in terms of systems biology, it should be highlighted that predictive medicine is necessarily evidence-based (Domenighetti et al. 1998; Hood and Flores 2012), and it is typically characterized by the usage of equations, formulas, and models to elaborate multiple variables in order to approximately describe future health-relevant events.

Medicine is **participatory** (cfr. Chap. 6) in that it does not operate in a social vacuum. Despite this, traditional medicine was perceived as an activity abstracted from the everyday social life of the patient, such as patient, doctor, and the disease interacted among themselves only (Gorini and Pravettoni 2011; Kabat-Zinn 2000). On the contrary, the process of care involves a number of additional stakeholders and influencers, such as caregivers, other patients, and different types of health providers (Gorini et al. 2018). This aspect of health should not only be made explicit but exploited, in that an effective alliance between the multiple actors of the care process is expected to strengthen its effectiveness.

As explained above, the 4 Ps in Leeroy Hood's model emerged from a conception rooted in systems biology and were then extended to social and ethical aspects. Doing so, the original model could not ignore another aspect which very much deserves to be included among its main pillars as well.

On this basis, recently Pravettoni and Gorini (Gorini and Pravettoni 2011; Pravettoni and Gorini 2011) proposed to add a fifth P to the model, namely, the **psychocognitive** one. Psychocognitive medicine (cfr. Chap. 7) emphasizes that the patient, considered as a person and not only as a recipient of care, is characterized by emotions, attitudes, and cognitive processes which have specific relations with his/her own care process. By embracing the fifth P, this approach has a conception of value in healthcare that goes beyond the evidence-based medicine approach (Marzorati and Pravettoni 2017; Riva and Pravettoni 2016); while evidence-based medicine is regarded as the results of clinical trials to identify the most desirable medical procedures and interventions, P5 considers the impact on quality of life as an additional fundamental marker of effectiveness.

Moreover, the fifth P has important methodological consequences for healthcare: future medicine should be able to design a psychological and cognitive profile of the patient, instead of a mere diagnostic classification; in this sense, P5 medicine leads to an assessment with psychometric tools that include cognitive, decision-making, and mental aspects, as well as clinical ones.

Specifically, to sum up, the fifth P proposes some activities to be considered fundamental in healthcare interventions (Pravettoni and Gorini 2011):

- Development and testing of new psychometric instruments, devoted to provide a complete medical profile of the patient.
- Promotion of the active patient's decision-making about therapy and healthcare process as a whole.
- The right for the patient to develop an empathic relationship with the physician.
- Assessment of quality of life and its inclusion among the criteria necessary to perform evaluation of clinical procedures and practices (value-based medicine).

For the sake of completeness, we could report that also a sixth P was proposed in the literature, namely, **public**; Bragazzi (2013) analyzed the famous case of Salvatore Iaconesi, a patient diagnosed with cancer who made his medical records available on the Internet and social media, inviting "everyone" to find a cure for his disease (not only in medical but also in emotional and spiritual terms). This case is interesting in that, according to Bragazzi, it shows how healthcare is evolving from a private and dyadic, paternalistic relationship between patient and physician to a public issue that extends the therapeutic alliance to multiple actors within the social context.

Anyway, this highlights again the importance of considering the patient as a whole person, not only a passive recipient of medical care but an active individual looking for meaning and personal actualization. Although some aspects of human experience (e.g., happiness, self-fulfillment, spirituality) should probably not be considered objectives of medicine, healthcare providers should take into account that patients with a chronic disease are not only combating a physical illness but also they are engaged in a personal journey whose final objective is the pursuit of happiness and fulfillment *besides or independently of* the presence of a chronic health condition.

Starting from these premises, healthcare providers of the future should be able to design, develop, and implement care projects and tools that, as first, do not prevent people to chase their own personal objectives but also, when possible, include affordances and opportunities to actively pursue them. New technologies could be a resource for such aims.

3 eHealth

In 2001, eHealth has been defined by Eysenbach (2001), who explained that the delivery of information to patients and stakeholders could be enriched by the intersection of medical informatics and public health business. On the other hand, he pointed out that not only a technical development is involved in the emergence of eHealth but also a new state of mind marked by a global-thinking attitude and by the intention to improve healthcare locally, regionally, and worldwide. In general, eHealth should be distinguished by medical informatics or the inclusion of computer and software in medical treatments and management, in order to improve care effectiveness: this discipline is way more "ancient" than eHealth; according to Mihalas and colleagues (2014), the history of medical informatics can be traced back before the 1970s, with pioneer work on signal analysis, modeling and simulation of biological processes, and the first attempts to develop decision support systems. It is around the 1980s that medical informatics acquired international recognition by means of funding, the development and sharing of methodologies, and the foundation of specialization schools. However, at the same time of the next generation in technology development, a first distinction is made between the use of computers for healthcare (to elaborate and process health-related information) to the communication features of technologies: this is the rise of "telehealth" and telemedicine" as concepts more focused on technological properties able to overcome boundaries and distances, this way promoting and strengthening communication between health providers and patients (Krol 1997; Palazzini 2007; Rubel et al. 2004; Wade et al. 2010).

In this context, eHealth should be considered another third evolution of the concept; according to Della Mea's editorial (Della Mea 2001), it could be considered the "death" of both medical informatics and telemedicine, in the sense that it encompasses them but also goes further and is more inclusive. Specifically, according to other opinions (Allen 2000; Rosen 2000), the focus of telemedicine was on hardware properties, while eHealth has a broader interest in how services are delivered; similarly, the "actors" of eHealth are the patients or better the health consumers, and not only the physicians or health providers. Reviews on eHealth definitions (Oh et al. 2005; Pagliari et al. 2005) highlighted that common aspects of different conceptions of eHealth still emphasize the usage of technologies for promoting healthcare, not only in terms of strictly clinical outcomes but also well-being and quality of life.

But what technologies should be considered typical of eHealth interventions? Actually, this question is not so easy to respond to; as what previously happened to other fields (such as "commerce"), the addition of "e" (electronic) referred to the use of the Internet and highlighted the new ways of performing activities, thanks to connection features represented by the web. This is certainly true for eHealth too, but some authors (Gorini et al. 2008; Riva 2000) also include in eHealth experiential technologies which are not connected to the Internet, such as Virtual Reality for the simulation and training of healthy behaviors and lifestyles. Conversely, others consider advanced "technical" technologies (i.e., for the analysis of clinical data and for supporting diagnosis, such as big data applications) examples of innovative eHealth applications (Luo et al. 2016).

According to a number of systematic reviews in the field (Barello et al. 2016; Black et al. 2011; Elbert et al. 2014), these appear to be the most frequent technologies used in eHealth interventions:

- **Informational websites**, that is, patients are given access to web resources that are either created or monitored by health providers, to guarantee reliable health information and promote health literacy.
- **Telecommunication technologies**, ranging from telephone to social media features, in order to improve communication between patients and the health providers.
- **Web platforms and "ePrescribing,"** bespoke web resources that include services for monitoring, signaling, and supporting treatment administration and adherence on patients' side.
- **Wearable technologies and mobile technology (*mHealth*)**, any use of portable technologies to monitor patients' health status over time and/or sending daily reminders to take medications or to perform health-related activities.
- **Online support groups**, social media for peer support and peer education (Gorini et al. 2018).

- **Decision support systems**, algorithm-based dedicated software that helps the physician and/or the patient to make decisions about the care path, by making explicit the possible choices and their consequences.

Other technologies appear considerably less often in eHealth literature but could be considered evolved tools, especially because they are based on more complex conceptions of technology's potential influence on users' everyday life and personal abilities. The design, development, and implementation of these technologies are often more expensive and require specific competences (Gorini et al. 2008; Riva 2000; Riva et al. 2006; Rizzo and Kim 2005; Triberti and Barello 2016; Triberti and Chirico 2016; Triberti et al. 2019):

- **Ambient Intelligence (AmI)**, which is an umbrella term identifying computers embedded in users' environment (e.g., the home) supporting everyday activities and health monitoring.
- **Video Games and Serious Games**, which proved to be effective both as training of abilities and health education and coping or stress/emotion management.
- (Immersive) **Virtual Reality**, usually for rehabilitation or relaxation purposes
- **Virtual Worlds**, internet-based two-dimensional or tridimensional virtual environments (that can be accessed by personal computer or mobile devices), explored by multiple users at a time, thanks to the use of digital avatars, including opportunities both for communication/peer support and for training/health education.
- **Robotics,** the employment of more-or-less humanlike robots to help patients, for example, assists them in life tasks when at home.

Consistently, Moen and colleagues (2013), who conducted surveys among national member associations of the European Federation of Medical Informatics (EFMI), classify eHealth services in three main categories:

- **Technical and social eHealth infrastructures**, namely, services for secure, seamless transmission of health information between home care/primary care, hospitals, and GPs and between public and private health.
- **eHealth repositories**, services that allow patients and health providers to securely access information and resources for coordination and self-management,
- **eHealth applications** (cfr. Chap. 4), specific services permitting communication between patients and health professionals.

A critical approach to the eHealth phenomenon requires recognizing its potentials but also its shortcomings; the next sections will explore the eHealth scenario in detail, in order to explain which aspects of healthcare technologies should be exploited or avoided in future implementations.

3.1 Strengths of eHealth

A number of studies explored positive aspects of eHealth, especially its effectiveness in improving physical (Norman et al. 2007; van den Berg et al. 2007) and psychological (Eland-de Kok et al. 2011) health outcomes.

Another fundamental aspect is related to cost-effectiveness or, better, the ability of eHealth interventions to reduce overall costs of managing disease and treatment in specific cases. Although methodological problems exist and there is always a quote of uncertainty in such evaluations (Bergmo 2015), data coming from simulations suggest that eHealth is able to sensibly reduce costs on healthcare systems (cfr. Chap. 4) (Smit et al. 2011; Stroetmann et al. 2006).

Additionally, it is well known that one of the main strengths of eHealth (and of telemedicine already) is its ability to overcome distances and periods of time (Drury 2005; Ray et al. 2015); for example, communication technologies for healthcare may be useful to reach patients living in rural areas and/or patients who, due to symptoms of their conditions or limited availability of caregivers, experience significant difficulties to move around places and so to reach medical facilities or other locations that are important for treatment adherence (e.g., rehabilitation, pharmacy, etc.).

For the same reason, eHealth and telemedicine permit "democratization" of patient-doctor communication and healthcare in general (Brandt et al. 2018; Brown et al. 2015), in that some health services could be made more accessible for everyone, more or less independently of the availability for the patient of economic resources.

eHealth is demonstrated to have a strong relation with engagement, on the one hand with *user* engagement, that is, patients are more likely to use technologies when these are designed to be pleasant, involving, or even funny (Craig Lefebvre et al. 2010; Graffigna et al. 2014); an example of this is the utilization of *gamification* or the inclusion of features typical of games and video games in health-related technological interfaces (McCallum 2012; Sardi et al. 2017); for instance, patients are invited to report their adherence behaviors such as their game achievements and the positive feedback and prizes they received.

On the other hand, eHealth has proven to promote *patient* engagement (Ahern et al. 2008; Barello et al. 2016), which is, as written above, patients' commitment to their own healthcare journey and ability to manage life commitments (e.g., work) despite illness (Riva et al. 2015). This is also related to the possibility for technology to promote knowledge/literacy and empower decision-making (Kondylakis et al. 2012, 2013; Norman and Skinner 2006; Wozney et al. 2017); indeed, information on health, therapy, and disease are made more accessible and easy to understand, and decisions to be taken may be represented and explained in the context of technology-enhanced decision support systems.

Finally, eHealth could provide opportunities to *structure* the participation to healthcare of multiple actors, not only patients and physicians but also caregivers, stakeholders, and multiple types of health providers; indeed, in the context of social media platforms, any figure important for patient's health and wellness could be his/her own profile and online presence, in order to actively and positively participate in the care process.

3.2 Criticalities of eHealth and Emerging Challenges

When considering eHealth, it is important to recognize also the shortcomings appearing in a number of technology implementation in healthcare and its possible risks and limitations.

One recent review (Granja et al. 2018) explored the factors determining success or failure of eHealth interventions: their results focused on category costs, specifically the authors highlighted that, from an organizational point of view, eHealth could enhance workload for healthcare professionals and cause workflow disruption, as well as complexify role definition and undermine face-to-face communication.

As abovementioned, eHealth is expected to reduce costs, but additional costs may develop regarding the technology design, maintenance, or possible redesign after negative results emerging from evaluation (Chaudhry et al. 2006). Consistently, the implementation of eHealth may require health providers to include additional, specific competences to make it work in the long run (e.g., technical assistance).

Moreover, although generally eHealth has potentialities in terms of user engagement, it should be recognized that patients and users in general may not have a positive attitude towards it (Currie et al. 2015; Légaré et al. 2010); *technology acceptance* is an important issue in this field, in that people may not be prone to actually use it, or sometimes they could even refuse to. Such behavior can be related to various forms of digital divide (Voelker 2001), for example, patients do not have (or think they have not) basic knowledge and competences in technology usage. It can also happen that users have an initial positive attitude towards technology, but they cease to use it after a given period of time; that is the reason why technology acceptance and technology adoption should be considered two separate issues, the last one pertaining to long-term usage and adherence to the system (Triberti et al. 2018). For this reason, the design of eHealth, and especially of its interfaces (i.e., the part of the technology which is in direct contact with the user), should be conducted giving high importance to usability and user experience, to the point that the gold standard for eHealth design is found by many authors in user-centered design (UCD) techniques cf. chapter 9 (Holzinger et al. 2009; Triberti and Barello 2016; Vorderstrasse et al. 2016). UCD refers to any design process where final users have an important influence on how the design itself takes place (Garrett 2010; Lowdermilk 2013); usually, this means employing qualitative research methods to analyze users' behavior, needs, and context to inform design and not only as a guide for evaluation, as it is done in the traditional usable approach. UCD may be costly as a first phase of an intervention, and also designers/engineers should be inclined to base their own work on the research data; however, when correctly applied, this approach could effectively eliminate usage issues that typically intervene at later stages of the intervention process.

Other important criticalities to consider in eHealth are related to privacy, in that various kinds of patients' data should be adequately preserved and protected, and ethics, because eHealth implementation should not become an excuse for physicians to "transfer" clinical care from themselves to software and machines; such an automatization of the healthcare process could be partly achieved, thanks to eHealth technologies, but could not be an objective for a patient-centered, P5-informed approach to patients and their illnesses.

4 Conclusion

This contribution briefly presented the P5 approach to medicine as an innovative perspective on how future medicine should evolve; numerous factors in patients' healthcare journey still have to mature in order to reach their full potentialities in terms of preventive, personalized, predictive, participatory, and psychocognitive properties. Taking this aim into consideration, we then proceeded to explore the concept of eHealth and its various incarnations in contemporary scientific literature; it has been shown how technologies for healthcare still hold tremendous potentialities to renovate the healthcare scenario globally, but also challenges and criticalities get in the way of progress.

For this reason, the subsequent contributions in the present book will explore a range of solutions to eHealth implementations issues, in order to give hints about the evolution of healthcare in general.

Five chapters will explore the 5 Ps one by one, focusing on guidelines for their implementations within technologies devoted to enhance the healthcare process; secondarily, other chapters will address specific issues such as the use for innovative technological resources for diagnosis, or common ethical dilemmas related to eHealth implementations.

References

Ahern, D., Phalen, J. M., & Eaton, C. B. (2008). The role of eHealth in patient engagement and quality improvement. In M. C. Gibbons (Ed.), *eHealth solutions for healthcare disparities* (pp. 75–92). Heidelberg: Springer. https://doi.org/10.1007/978-0-387-72815-5_9.

Allen, A. (2000). Morphing telemedicine – telecare – telehealth – eHealth. *Telemedicine Today, 1*, 43.

Anderson, R. M., & Funnell, M. M. (2010). Patient empowerment: Myths and misconceptions. *Patient Education and Counseling, 79*(3), 277–282. https://doi.org/10.1016/j.pec.2009.07.025.

Balint, M., Hunt, J., Joyce, D., & Marinker, M. (1970). *Treatment or diagnosis: A study of repeat prescriptions in general practice*. London: Routledge.

Bardes, C. L. (2012). Defining "patient-centered medicine". *New England Journal of Medicine, 366*(9), 782–783. https://doi.org/10.1056/NEJMp1200070.

Barello, S., Graffigna, G., & Vegni, E. (2012). Patient engagement as an emerging challenge for healthcare services: Mapping the literature. *Nursing Research and Practice, 2012*, 1–7. https://doi.org/10.1155/2012/905934.

Barello, S., Triberti, S., Graffigna, G., Libreri, C., Serino, S., Hibbard, J. H., & Riva, G. (2016). eHealth for patient engagement: A systematic review. *Frontiers in Psychology, 6*, 2013. https://doi.org/10.3389/fpsyg.2015.02013.

Bergmo, T. S. (2015). How to measure costs and benefits of ehealth interventions: An overview of methods and frameworks. *Journal of Medical Internet Research*. https://doi.org/10.2196/jmir.4521.

Black, A. D., Car, J., Pagliari, C., Anandan, C., Cresswell, K., Bokun, T., … Sheikh, A. (2011). The impact of ehealth on the quality and safety of health care: A systematic overview. *PLoS Medicine, 8*(1). https://doi.org/10.1371/journal.pmed.1000387.

Bragazzi, N. L. (2013). From P0 to P6 medicine, a model of highly participatory, narrative, interactive, and "augmented" medicine: Some considerations on Salvatore Iaconesi's clinical story. *Patient Preference and Adherence, 7*, 353–359. https://doi.org/10.2147/PPA.S38578.

Brandt, J. C., Sogaard, I. G., Clemensen, J., Sndergaard, J., & Nielsen, B. J. (2018). General practitioners? Perspective on eHealth and lifestyle change: Qualitative interview study. *JMIR mHealth and uHealth, 6*(4), e88. https://doi.org/10.2196/mhealth.8988.

Brown, P., Elston, M. A., & Gabe, J. (2015). From patient deference towards negotiated and precarious informality: An Eliasian analysis of English general practitioners' understandings of changing patient relations. *Social Science and Medicine, 146*, 164–172. https://doi.org/10.1016/j.socscimed.2015.10.047.

Cesario, A., Auffray, C., Russo, P., & Hood, L. (2014). P4 medicine needs P4 education. *Current Pharmaceutical Design, 20*(38), 6071–6072. https://doi.org/10.2174/1381612820666140314145445.

Chaudhry, B., Wang, J., Wu, S., Maglione, M., Mojica, W., Roth, E., … Shekelle, P. G. (2006). Systematic review: Impact of health information technology on quality, efficiency, and costs of medical care. *Annals of Internal Medicine, 144*(10), 742–752. https://doi.org/0000605-200605160-00125[pii]

Craig Lefebvre, R., Tada, Y., Hilfiker, S. W., & Baur, C. (2010). The assessment of user engagement with eHealth content: The eHealth engagement scale. *Journal of Computer-Mediated Communication, 15*(4), 666–681. https://doi.org/10.1111/j.1083-6101.2009.01514.x.

Currie, M., Philip, L. J., & Roberts, A. (2015). Attitudes towards the use and acceptance of eHealth technologies: A case study of older adults living with chronic pain and implications for rural healthcare. *BMC Health Services Research, 15*(1), 162. https://doi.org/10.1186/s12913-015-0825-0.

Cutica, I., Vie, G. M., & Pravettoni, G. (2014). Personalised medicine: The cognitive side of patients. *European Journal of Internal Medicine, 25*(8), 685–688. https://doi.org/10.1016/j.ejim.2014.07.002.

Della Mea, V. (2001). What is e-health (2): The death of telemedicine? *Journal of Medical Internet Research, 3*(2), 6–7. https://doi.org/10.2196/jmir.3.2.e22.

Domenighetti, G., Grilli, R., & Liberati, A. (1998). Promoting consumers' demand for evidence-based medicine. *International Journal of Technology Assessment in Health Care*. https://doi.org/10.1017/S0266462300010552.

Drury, P. (2005). The eHealth agenda for developing countries. *World Hospitals and Health Services, 41*(4), 38–40. Retrieved from http://www.ncbi.nlm.nih.gov/pubmed/16512063.

Eisen, M. B., Spellman, P. T., Brown, P. O., & Botstein, D. (1998). Cluster analysis and display of genome-wide expression patterns. *Proceedings of the National Academy of Sciences of the United States of America, 95*(25), 14863–14868. https://doi.org/10.1073/pnas.95.25.14863.

Eland-de Kok, P., van Os-Medendorp, H., Vergouwe-Meijer, A., Bruijnzeel-Koomen, C., & Ros, W. (2011). A systematic review of the effects of e-health on chronically ill patients. *Journal of Clinical Nursing*. https://doi.org/10.1111/j.1365-2702.2011.03743.x.

Elbert, N. J., van Os-Medendorp, H., van Renselaar, W., Ekeland, A. G., Hakkaart-van Roijen, L., Raat, H., … Pasmans, S. G. M. A. (2014). Effectiveness and cost-effectiveness of ehealth interventions in somatic diseases: A systematic review of systematic reviews and meta-analyses. *Journal of Medical Internet Research, 16*(4), e110. https://doi.org/10.2196/jmir.2790.

Eysenbach, G. (2001). What is e-health? *Journal of Medical Internet Research, 3*, e22. https://doi.org/10.2196/jmir.3.2.e20.

Fioretti, C., Mazzocco, K., Riva, S., Oliveri, S., Masiero, M., & Pravettoni, G. (2016). Research studies on patients' illness experience using the narrative medicine approach: A systematic review. *BMJ Open, 6*(7), e011220.

Garrett, J. J. (2010). *Elements of user experience, the: User-centered design for the web and beyond* (Pearson ed.). Berkeley: Pearson Education.

Gorini, A., & Pravettoni, G. (2011). P5 medicine: A plus for a personalized approach to oncology. *Nature Reviews Clinical Oncology*. https://doi.org/10.1038/nrclinonc.2010.227-c1.

Gorini, A., Gaggioli, A., Vigna, C., & Riva, G. (2008). A second life for eHealth: Prospects for the use of 3-D virtual worlds in clinical psychology. *Journal of Medical Internet Research, 10*, e21. https://doi.org/10.2196/jmir.1029.

Gorini, A., Mazzocco, K., Triberti, S., Sebri, V., Savioni, L., & Pravettoni, G. (2018). A P5 approach to m-health: Development guidelines for advanced mobile health technology. *Frontiers in Psychology, 9*, 2066. https://doi.org/10.3389/fpsyg.2018.02066.

Graffigna, G., Barello, S., Triberti, S., Wiederhold, B. K., Bosio, A. C., & Riva, G. (2014). Enabling eHealth as a pathway for patient engagement: A toolkit for medical practice. *Studies in Health Technology and Informatics, 199*, 13–21. Retrieved from http://www.ncbi.nlm.nih.gov/pubmed/24875682.

Graffigna, G., Barello, S., & Triberti, S. (2016). *Patient engagement: A consumer-centered model to innovate healthcare*. Berlin: De Gruyter Open.

Granja, C., Janssen, W., & Johansen, M. A. (2018). Factors determining the success and failure of eHealth interventions: Systematic review of the literature corresponding author. *Journal of Medical Internet Research, 20*, 1–21. https://doi.org/10.2196/10235.

Hanyok, L. A., Hellmann, D. B., Rand, C., & Ziegelstein, R. C. (2012). Practicing patient-centered care: The questions clinically excellent physicians use to get to know their patients as individuals. *Patient, 5*(3), 141–145. https://doi.org/10.2165/11599530.

Hibbard, J. H., Mahoney, E. R., Stock, R., & Tusler, M. (2007). Do increases in patient activation result in improved self-management behaviors? *Health Services Research, 42*, 1443–1463. https://doi.org/10.1111/j.1475-6773.2006.00669.x.

Holzinger, A., Miesenberger, K., Gaul, S., & Ziefle, M. (2009). HCI and usability for e-inclusion. *Lecture Notes in Computer Science, 5889*(November 2009), 312–332. https://doi.org/10.1007/978-3-642-10308-7.

Hood, L. (2009). Systems medicine, transformational technologies and the emergence of predictive, personalized, preventive and participatory (P4) medicine. In *Proceedings of the conference on high performance computing networking, storage and analysis – SC '09* (p. 2). https://doi.org/10.1145/1654059.1657026

Hood, L. (2013). Systems biology and P4 medicine: Past, present, and future. *Rambam Maimonides Medical Journal, 4*(2), e0012. https://doi.org/10.5041/RMMJ.10112.

Hood, L., & Flores, M. (2012). A personal view on systems medicine and the emergence of proactive P4 medicine: Predictive, preventive, personalized and participatory. *New Biotechnology, 29*(6), 613–624. https://doi.org/10.1016/j.nbt.2012.03.004.

Hood, L. E., & Galas, D. J. (2008). P4 *medicine: Personalized, predictive, preventive, participatory a change of view that changes everything*. A white paper prepared for the Computing Community Consortium committee of the Computing Research Association. http://cra.org/ccc/resources/ccc-led-whitepapers/

Kabat-Zinn, J. (2000). Participatory medicine. *Journal of the European Academy of Dermatology and Venereology*. https://doi.org/10.1046/j.1468-3083.2000.00062.x.

Kondylakis, H., Koumakis, L., Genitsaridi, E., Tsiknakis, M., Marias, K., Pravettoni, G., … Mazzocco, K. (2012). IEmS: A collaborative environment for patient empowerment. In *IEEE 12th International conference on bioinformatics and bioengineering, BIBE 2012* (pp. 535–540). https://doi.org/10.1109/BIBE.2012.6399770

Kondylakis, H., Koumakis, L., Tsiknakis, M., Marias, K., Genitsaridi, E., Pravettoni, G., … Mazzocco, K. (2013). Smart recommendation services in support of patient empowerment and personalized medicine. *Smart Innovation, Systems and Technologies*. https://doi.org/10.1007/978-3-319-00375-7_4.

Krol, M. (1997). Telemedicine. *IEEE Potentials*. https://doi.org/10.1109/45.624339.

Légaré, F., Ratté, S., Stacey, D., Kryworuchko, J., Gravel, K., Graham, I. D., & Turcotte, S. (2010). Interventions for improving the adoption of shared decision making by healthcare professionals. *Cochrane Database of Systematic Reviews (Online)*, CD006732. https://doi.org/10.1002/14651858.CD006732.pub2.

Levenstein, J. H. (1984). The patient-centred general practice consultation. *South African Family Practice, 5*, 276–282.

Liberati, E. G., Gorli, M., Moja, L., Galuppo, L., Ripamonti, S., & Scaratti, G. (2015). Exploring the practice of patient centered care: The role of ethnography and reflexivity. *Social Science and Medicine, 133*, 45–52. https://doi.org/10.1016/j.socscimed.2015.03.050.

Lowdermilk, T. (2013). *User-centered design: A developer's guide to building user-friendly applications*. Sebastopol: O'Reilly.

Luo, J., Wu, M., Gopukumar, D., & Zhao, Y. (2016). Big data application in biomedical research and health care: A literature review. *Biomedical Informatics Insights, 8*, 1–10. https://doi.org/10.4137/BII.S31559.

Marzorati, C., & Pravettoni, G. (2017). Value as the key concept in the health care system: How it has influenced medical practice and clinical decision-making processes. *Journal of Multidisciplinary Healthcare, 10*, 101–106. https://doi.org/10.2147/JMDH.S122383.

McCallum, S. (2012). Gamification and serious games for personalized health. *Studies in Health Technology and Informatics, 177*, 85–96. https://doi.org/10.3233/978-1-61499-069-7-85.

Mihalas, G., Zvarova, J., Kulikowski, C., Ball, M., Bemmel, J., Hasman, A., … Barber, B. (2014). History of medical informatics in Europe – a short review by different approach. *Acta Informatica Medica, 22*(1), 6. https://doi.org/10.5455/aim.2014.22.6-10

Miller, D., Steele Gray, C., Kuluski, K., & Cott, C. (2015). Patient-centered care and patient-reported measures: Let's look before we leap. *Patient, 8*(4), 293–299. https://doi.org/10.1007/s40271-014-0095-7.

Moen, A., Hackl, W. O., Hofdijk, J., Van Gemert-Pijnen, L., Ammenwerth, E., Nykänen, P., & Hoerbst, A. (2013). eHealth in Europe – Status and challenges. *Yearbook of Medical Informatics, 22*(01), 59–63. https://doi.org/10.1055/s-0038-1638833.

Nicolini, C., Bragazzi, N., & Pechkova, E. (2012). Nanoproteomics enabling personalized nanomedicine. *Advanced Drug Delivery Reviews*. https://doi.org/10.1016/j.addr.2012.06.015.

Norman, C. D., & Skinner, H. A. (2006). eHealth literacy: Essential skills for consumer health in a networked world. *Journal of Medical Internet Research*. https://doi.org/10.2196/jmir.8.2.e9.

Norman, G. J., Zabinski, M. F., Adams, M. A., Rosenberg, D. E., Yaroch, A. L., & Atienza, A. A. (2007). A review of eHealth interventions for physical activity and dietary behavior change. *American Journal of Preventive Medicine*. https://doi.org/10.1016/j.amepre.2007.05.007.

Oh, H., Rizo, C., Enkin, M., Jadad, A., Powell, J., & Pagliari, C. (2005). What is eHealth (3): A systematic review of published definitions. *Journal of Medical Internet Research, 7*(1), e1. https://doi.org/10.2196/jmir.7.1.e1.

Pagliari, C., Sloan, D., Gregor, P., Sullivan, F., Detmer, D., Kahan, J. P., … MacGillivray, S. (2005). What is eHealth (4): A scoping exercise to map the field. *Journal of Medical Internet Research, 7*, e9. https://doi.org/10.2196/jmir.7.1.e9.

Palazzini, G. (2007). Telemedicine. *Il Giornale di Chirurgia, 28*(5), 232–234.

Pravettoni, G. (2016). Empowerment-based holistic cancer care. *Psycho-Oncology, 25*(Supple), 165.

Pravettoni, G., & Gorini, A. (2011). A P5 cancer medicine approach: Why personalized medicine cannot ignore psychology. *Journal of Evaluation in Clinical Practice, 17*(4), 594–596. https://doi.org/10.1111/j.1365-2753.2011.01709.x.

Pulciani, S., Di Lonardo, A., Fagnani, C., & Taruscio, D. (2017). P4 medicine versus Hippocrates. *Annali Dell'Istituto Superiore Della Sanità, 53*(3), 185–191. https://doi.org/10.4415/ANN_17_03_02.

Ray, K. N., Demirci, J. R., Bogen, D. L., Mehrotra, A., & Miller, E. (2015). Optimizing telehealth strategies for subspecialty care: Recommendations from rural pediatricians. *TeleMedicine and EHealth, 21*(8), 622–629. https://doi.org/10.1089/tmj.2014.0186.

Remmers, C., Hibbard, J., Mosen, D. M., Wagenfield, M., Hoye, R. E., & Jones, C. (2009). Is patient activation associated with future health outcomes and healthcare utilization among patients with diabetes? *The Journal of Ambulatory Care Management, 32*(4), 320–327. https://doi.org/10.1097/JAC.0b013e3181ba6e77.

Renzi, C., Riva, S., Masiero, M., & Pravettoni, G. (2016). The choice dilemma in chronic hematological conditions: Why choosing is not only a medical issue? A psycho-cognitive perspective. *Critical Reviews in Oncology/Hematology*. https://doi.org/10.1016/j.critrevonc.2015.12.010.

Renzi, C., Fioretti, C., Oliveri, S., Mazzocco, K., Zerini, D., Alessandro, O., … Pravettoni, G. (2017). A qualitative investigation on patient empowerment in prostate cancer. *Frontiers in Psychology, 8*(July), 1215. https://doi.org/10.3389/fpsyg.2017.01215.

Riva, G. (2000). From telehealth to E-health: Internet and distributed virtual reality in health care. *CyberPsychology and Behavior*. https://doi.org/10.1089/109493100452255.

Riva, S., & Pravettoni, G. (2016). Value-based model: A new perspective in medical decision-making. *Frontiers in Public Health, 4*, 118. https://doi.org/10.3389/fpubh.2016.00118.

Riva, G., Castelnuovo, G., & Mantovani, F. (2006). Transformation of flow in rehabilitation: The role of advanced communication technologies. *Behavior Research Methods, 38*(2), 237–244.

Riva, S., Cutica, I., Krampe, C., Reinecke, L. F., Russell-Edu, W., Santoro, C., … Pravettoni, G. (2015). A cohort pilot study on HIV-associated neuropsychological impairments in hemophilia patients. *Frontiers in Human Neuroscience, 9*, 313.

Rizzo, A. A., & Kim, G. J. (2005). A SWOT analysis of the field of virtual reality rehabilitation and therapy. *Presence: Teleoperators and Virtual Environments, 14*(2), 119–146. https://doi.org/10.1162/1054746053967094.

Rosen, E. (2000). The death of telemedicine? *Telemedicine Today, 8*(1), 14–17.

Rubel, P., Fayn, J., Simon-Chautemps, L., Atoui, H., Ohlsson, M., Telisson, D., … Chevalier, P. (2004). New paradigms in telemedicine: Ambient intelligence, wearable, pervasive and personalized. In *Wearable eHealth systems for personalised health management: State of the art and future challenges* (Vol. 108). Fairfax: IOS Press.

Sardi, L., Idri, A., & Fernández-Alemán, J. L. (2017). A systematic review of gamification in e-Health. *Journal of Biomedical Informatics*. https://doi.org/10.1016/j.jbi.2017.05.011.

Smit, F., Lokkerbol, J., Riper, H., Majo, M. C., Boon, B., & Blankers, M. (2011). Modeling the cost-effectiveness of health care systems for alcohol use disorders: How implementation of eHealth interventions improves cost-effectiveness. *Journal of Medical Internet Research, 13*(3), e56. https://doi.org/10.2196/jmir.1694.

Stroetmann, K. A., Jones, T., Dobrev, A., & Stroetmann, V. N. (2006). *eHealth is Worth it. eHealth Impact*. https://doi.org/10.2759/242.

Triberti, S., & Barello, S. (2016). The quest for engaging AmI: Patient engagement and experience design tools to promote effective assisted living. *Journal of Biomedical Informatics, 63*. https://doi.org/10.1016/j.jbi.2016.08.010.

Triberti, S., & Chirico, A. (2016). Healthy avatars, healthy people. In G. Graffigna (Ed.), *Transformative healthcare practice through patient engagement* (pp. 247–275). Hersey: IGI Global. https://doi.org/10.4018/978-1-5225-0663-8.ch010.

Triberti, S., Kelders, S. M., & Gaggioli, A. (2018). User Engagement. In L. van Gemert-Pijnen, S. Kelders, H. Kip, & R. Sanderman (Eds.), *eHealth research, theory and development*. Routledge.

Triberti, S., Gorini, A., Savioni, L., Sebri, V., & Pravettoni, G. (2019). Avatars and the disease: Digital customization as a resource for self-perception assessment in breast Cancer patients. *Cyberpsychology, Behavior and Social Networking, 22*(8), 558–564.

van den Berg, M. H., Schoones, J. W., & Vliet Vlieland, T. P. M. (2007). Internet-based physical activity interventions: A systematic review of the literature. *Journal of Medical Internet Research, 9*, e26. https://doi.org/10.2196/jmir.9.3.e26.

Voelker, R. (2001). Bridging the digital divide. *JAMA: The Journal of the American Medical Association, 285*(2), 156-c-156. https://doi.org/10.1001/jama.285.2.156-c.

Vorderstrasse, A., Lewinski, A., Melkus, G. D., & Johnson, C. (2016). Social support for diabetes self-management via eHealth interventions. *Current Diabetes Reports*. https://doi.org/10.1007/s11892-016-0756-0.

Wade, V. A., Karnon, J., Elshaug, A. G., & Hiller, J. E. (2010). A systematic review of economic analyses of telehealth services using real time video communication. *BMC Health Services Research, 10*, 233. https://doi.org/10.1186/1472-6963-10-233.

Wozney, L., Newton, A. S., Gehring, N. D., Bennett, K., Huguet, A., Hartling, L., … McGrath, P. (2017). Implementation of eMental health care: Viewpoints from key informants from organizations and agencies with eHealth mandates. *BMC Medical Informatics and Decision Making, 17*(1). https://doi.org/10.1186/s12911-017-0474-9.

Chapter 2
The Development of iManageCancer: The Experience of a Personalised eHealth Platform for Cancer Patients' Empowerment

Chiara Crico and Chiara Renzi

1 Introduction

According to Fleming and colleagues (Fleming et al. 2016), the traditional randomised clinical trial approach may be problematic for the testing of eHealth interventions due to the speed of technology change. They state that alternative models of rapid development and iterative testing should be considered (cfr. Chap. 9), for example, using AGILE software design principles, such as the lean start-up method (Nobel 2011) or scrum (Schwaber and Beedle 2002). In AGILE development processes, the product is tested with users from the outset using rapid development and testing feedback loops. An important component involves the development of a minimal viable product (MVP). A MVP is a barely finished product that contains an essential element, with missing details, and is provided to end-users to gage their reactions and inform the next steps in development. Reponses to the product are measured and used to inform next steps that are rapidly developed and tested in the same way. This iterative process involves close collaboration between designers, software developers, and end-users. Larger-scale testing gradually replaces small opportunistic samples as progressively more complex features are tested. When a near-finished version is ready, more traditional testing can be carried out, for example, via a randomised controlled trial. As described by Mohr et al. (1994), Internet interventions can utilise approaches that focus on evaluating the working mechanisms, rather than a locked-down version of the intervention. Such a framework allows for improvements in functionality to be made during a trial, subsequently resulting in a more generalisable and durable intervention (Favrod and Khazaal 2018).

C. Crico (✉)
Department of Oncology and Hemato-Oncology, University of Milan, Milan, Italy
e-mail: chiara.crico@unimi.it

C. Renzi
Applied Research Division for Cognitive and Psychological Science,
European Institute of Oncology IRCCS, Milan, Italy

G. Pravettoni, S. Triberti (eds.), *P5 eHealth: An Agenda for the Health Technologies of the Future*, https://doi.org/10.1007/978-3-030-27994-3_2

In accordance with this approach, the iManageCancer platform has been tested already by 19 of end-users as a result of the previous works of the project. Following the feedbacks received, the platform went through major updates and improvements, to get the platform ready for clinical context and to better assess its efficacy (Kondylakis et al. 2017).

2 The IManageCancer Platform

The iManageCancer platform is a set of interconnected health apps and games intended to empower patients with cancer and to support them in the management of their disease. Figure 2.1 illustrates the overall structure of the iManageCancer platform to be tested in the pilot. The platform comprises three apps and a serious game for adult cancer patients (see Fig. 2.1). Basic characteristics of these apps are shown in Fig. 2.2 followed by an explanation of the intended purpose of these apps. All apps operate on a common backbone of the platform that contains the data store with the patients' personal health records, the security and access control services,

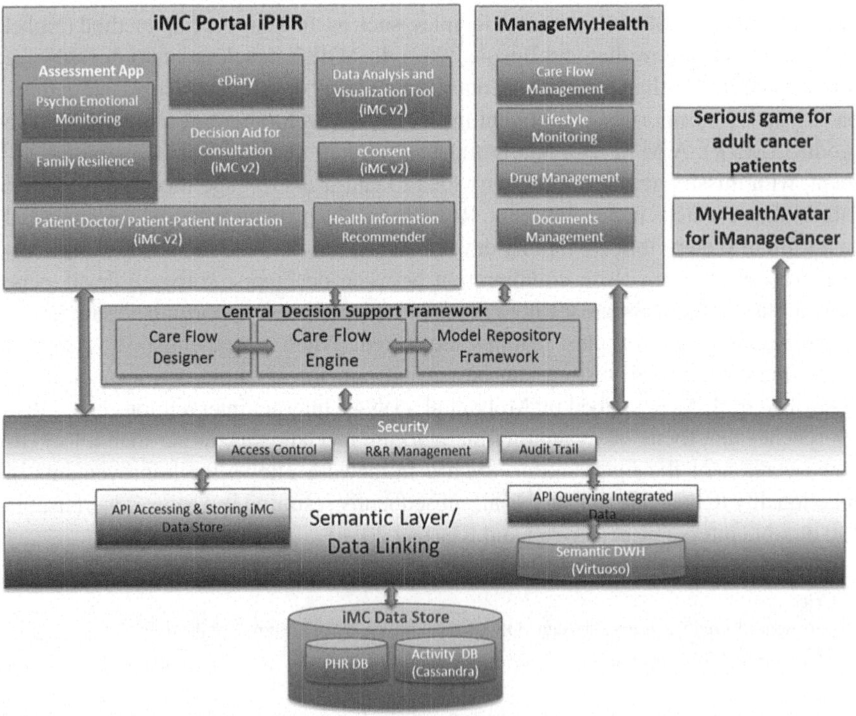

Fig. 2.1 High-level architecture of initial iManageCancer platform prototype. The applications shown with a blue background will be provided to the subjects of this pilot

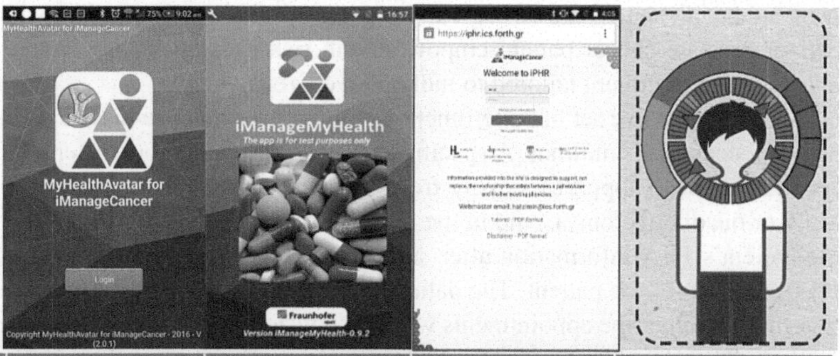

	University of Bedfordshire	Fraunhofer Gesellschaft	FORTH	University of Bedfordshire
Users	patients	patients	patients, doctors, researchers	Patients
Devices	Android 5, 6	Android 5, 6	Web app: all	Android, iOS
Gadgets	actimeters, scale	scale, BPM, thermometer		
Intended purpose	life style management for prostate and breast cancer patients	general health management	health management	Education
Integra-ted tools	Suites for weight, diet, activity, sleep, emotion, exercises, medication, questionnaires, and journal	drug management, vital signs monitoring, documents management, pain management	eDiary and PHR, data sharing, Health information Recommender, psycho-emotional monitoring	

Fig. 2.2 Overview about the different end-user applications of the iManageCancer platform that will be used in this clinical investigation

and also a central decision support framework. The latter provides for this pilot information services for patients for the management of side effects of cancer therapies such as pain and fatigue.

The following sections briefly present each of the applications and the game with their intended purpose and their main characteristics.

2.1 My HealthAvatar for iManageCancer

MyHealthAvatar for iManageCancer is a solution to support patients with prostate cancer and breast cancer to optimise their lifestyle and to recover from cancer treatment. The app offers access, collection, and sharing of long-term and consistent personal health status data through an integrated digital representation, which helps deliver prostate cancer patient empowerment, risk prediction, prevention, clinical analysis, and treatment tailored to individual citizens.

A comprehensive set of suite functions let the user manage his/her weight, diet, activity, sleep, and emotions. A specific exercise suite offers four different exercises for the patient to support recovery from prostatectomy or breast surgery (mastectomy or quadrantectomy). And in the man's version, a Questionnaire Suite collects the patient's PSA information after surgery in order to let the doctor monitor the PSA changes for the patient. The patient can create alarms in the Medication Suite to remind him/her the appointments with the physician or to take a drug. A calendar feature allows him/her to easily schedule such events. A journal provides cancer-related health tips and selected health information. A pain and emotion monitor is used to collect the patient's mood and emotion information. The questionnaire of mood and emotion appears three times a day in the journal page. The patient can also set lifestyle-related goals, including weight monitoring, diet, or physical activity. A daily summary displays the daily/weekly/monthly results of the measured values comparing to the goals and reminders that help the patient to achieve his/her goals. The patient can also enable location tracking and check the daily location and tracking path in the app. Patient can annotate the places he/she visited which will be synchronized to the server. Furthermore, the patient can edit his/her health profile and share this information with other users of the app if he/she wants. And in the man's version, A Questionnaire Suite collects the patient's PSA information after surgery in order to let the doctor monitor the PSA changes for the patient.

2.2 *iManageMyHealth*

iManageMyHealth is a multipurpose informative app intended for citizens and patients for general health management. It supports users (1) in managing their drugs and drug intakes, also by providing a reminder system to facilitate adherence to treatment; (2) in providing information on drugs and their interactions; (3) in managing and understanding their paper-based health documents; and (4) in recording and overviewing specific vital signs and laboratory parameters.

Further, the app also provides specific management services in the context of cancer, as for the record of felt level of pain and the link to public information resources. The app as a whole is not intended for diagnosis and therapy but just as a supportive electronic solution for information provision and management of medical information.The following functionality is offered for the management of drugs:

- Add a new drug to the medication plan. When patients start to enter the medication name, an autocomplete feature proposes drugs with the help of one of the two external drug information services. The user is encouraged to take pictures of the drug package and the drug itself. Furthermore, he can specify drug intake times. The system reminds him with a message to take the drug. There is also space for personal comments to the drugs. Information on a new drug in the medication plan is also sent to the iPHR (see description below).

- The new drug is checked for potential interactions with other drugs in the medication plan (if the drugs are known to the external drug information service). Warning symbols are shown in the medication plan, and drug-drug interaction information is presented when the user touches the warning symbol. This feature is only offered in the German and English version of the app, as it relies on external national drug information services and their capabilities.
- Delete a drug from the medication plan. All information related to the drug is deleted from the system, and the patient is asked about its effectiveness. This information is also sent to iPHR.
- More information about a drug is shown by forwarding the user to the webpage https://www.drugs.com/ containing structured information about the drug (in English language only).
- This component leverages the Canadian Internet-based drug information service DrugBank of OMx Personal Health Analytics Inc. to select drugs from a list, to present information on drugs, and to check contraindications. The Canadian DrugBank does not only contain approved drugs for the US and Canadian market but also includes drugs registered at EMA for the European market. However, as brand names of the different drugs may differ in Italy, the Italian drug information tables "Lista farmaci di classe A e H per consentire a tutti gli Operatori la prescrizione per principio attivo" published on http://www.aifa.gov.it/content/dati-sulle-liste-dei-farmaci-open-data is used in the Italian version of the app instead. In order to counterbalance the risk of patients self-adjusting drug intakes, the app contains a disclaimer which specifies that the app does not constitute or substitute a medical consultation and that changes to the medication plan should always be discussed with the treating physician(s).

The following functionality is offered for managing health documents:

The app offers the user to scan paper-based health documents and to store them in the Android device and to annotate them. Scanning is done with the camera, and a document is assembled as a set of images. The user can go through a document page by page and can zoom in and out in a page. He can mark a section with a keyword and search with this marked text in Wikipedia or in the Personal Health Information Recommender. Results are presented to the user.

The following functionality is offered for monitoring vital signs and lab parameters:

- The patient can enter results of blood pressure readings, his weight, and his body temperatures. The values are presented in charts.
- The patient can enter lab results of the blood parameters PSA, leucocytes, and neutrophils.

2.3 iManageCancer Portal iPHR

The iPHR enables an individual to own and manage a complete, secure, digital copy of his/her health and wellness information. It integrates health information across sites of care and over time. The system is essentially an inversion of the current approach to medical records, in that the record resides with the patients and the patients grant permissions to institutions, clinicians, researchers, and other users of medical information. iPHR is a distributed, web-based, personally controlled electronic medical record system that is ubiquitously accessible to the nomadic user, built to public standards.

The iPHR is composed of many applications including:

- eDiary – Calendar: A timeline view of all available information showing medications, problems, appointments, and procedures.
- Demographics: View and update patient information such as gender, date of birth, contact information, name, and surname.
- Labs: View and update laboratory result values.
- Problems: View and update diseases, illnesses, injuries, and physiologic, mental, or psychological condition or disorders.
- Procedures: View and update medical treatments or operations of the patient.
- Allergies: View and update abnormal reactions to encountered allergens.
- Medications: View and update drugs or other substances received.
- Measurements: View and update vital signs that indicate the status of the body's vital functions.
- Contact: A form to communicate with other users of the system.
- Appointments: View and update appointments between the patient and doctors.
- Upload Documents: Upload your health data documents.
- Psychoemotional and health assessment tools.
- Personal Health Information Recommender: Allow patients to search in a high-quality document repository for useful information.

2.4 Game for Adults

The aim of the serious game is to promote self-efficacy, i.e. the belief of the patients to be able to manage and face their disease, also to help the patient deal with the psychological dimension of their disease, and to promote a healthier lifestyle and disease management. The serious game for adults puts the user in the role of an authority figure who manages a small town where they help residents with their cancer-related lifestyle problems. The user is invited to think critically and strategically in order to balance their resources and time, while also viewing the issues surrounding their cancer from a different perspective. The game is intended to promote the concept that a good management of a person's cancer disease is possible, together with the achievement of a sense of wellbeing.

The serious game's implementation is a full 3D simulation utilising the unity 3D platform and running on Android mobile devices. The game world itself is a colourful and stylised representation of a town, providing an environment for the user's avatar to exist and interact with town services and other characters. The game provides an easy-to-use social interface to allow users to make and manage friends. The serious game also links into the iMC back end services in order to leverage a user's personal activity as an in-game resource. Users can also customise their avatar's appearance and clothing using the simple character builder and in-game item store. The game avoids making recommendations about the user's real cancer disease; instead, the game attempts to provide generalised knowledge related to health and lifestyle through the trivia mini-game and the instructions given to the simulated cancer patient (not the user) by the in-game doctor.

3 iManageCancer Within the p5 Approach

The iManageCancer project is a good example of how an eHealth intervention can be integrated with the properties of the P5 medicine towards the improvement of patient empowerment and quality of life: the following paragraphs will give an overview on how eHealth-based projects can lead medical practice towards a preventive, personalised, predictive, participatory, and psychocognitive approach (Pravettoni and Gorini 2011).

The multiple monitoring functions of the iManageCancer platform act as a *preventive*, according to its definition as the ability to proactively address diseases. Some of the apps are meant to give patients and clinicians the possibility to achieve a complete medical profile of patients and easily monitor their quality of life, by assessing both psychological and physical condition. In the iPHR, patients are provided with a set of three questionnaires to assess psychological wellbeing by measuring factors that play an important role in the care path. The questionnaires are ALGA, developed to assess physical and mental characteristics of cancer patients (Gorini et al. 2015); a psychoemotional monitoring tool; and FaRe, a questionnaire to assess the family resilience (Faccio et al. 2018). Moreover, the MyHealthAvatar (Zhang et al. 2018) is an activity tracker and a lifestyle monitoring app: it keeps track of sleep, weight, diet, sedentary lifestyle, and motor activities. The app promotes a good lifestyle and encourages healthy habits by helping patients manage their activities; it also monitors psychological status by proving a journal and a mood state to be updated every day from patients. In addition, the three questionnaires give an insight about the psychological status of patients and monitor potential changes in their mental wellbeing. Thanks to all these features, the platform that provides health professionals – both physicians and psychologists – with real-time data allows capturing any situation at risk and intervening in advance in order to address potential pathologies and provide patients with the necessary medical or psychological support.

As we have seen in the detailed description of the apps, many of their internal functions have been conceived as containers in which patients can insert all the specific information of their personal state: from the average information, such as values and findings, to the details of their lifestyle and habits and from the emotional and psychological status to their decision preferences. All the contents in this virtual database create a personalised profile of the patient, which can be used as a basis for a tailored intervention. For instance, the iPHR provides the psychological questionnaires to assess not only physical but also mental health degeneration and social alienation and to provide personalised information for coping strategies. Even the iManageMyHealth app is totally customisable, helping patients manage the variety of their drugs, prescribed by different factors for different clinical conditions and comorbidities. It acts as a container for all medical reports and prescriptions, and patients can insert the drugs they are taking, including time and mode of intake. This app is programmed to give back personalised information as output, including potential integrations among drugs and predictable side effects related to their clinical condition. A comprehensive consideration of all this aspects, which go beyond the mere biological information, points towards a more *personalised* medicine (Cutica et al. 2014; Renzi et al. 2016), as described in the P5 model. Also, the application contains specific features, such as the digital avatar to represent the user and his/her own health state, which could be important for personalisation in terms of self-expression (cfr. Chap. 4).

Putting together the advances of systems biology in the diagnostic field with the potential of the technological tools available today opens up new scenarios and increasingly important challenges for eHealth to predict the onset of pathological events. Considering that the exploitation of ICT in all its forms is, in this field, a recent development, one of the objectives of iManageCancer has been (Kim et al. 2018) to develop and incorporate in the platform *predictive* models for the early detection of severe adverse reaction to chemotherapy, in order to increase patients safety and wellbeing.

The general aim of the iManageCancer project is to empower patients by giving them tools to gain a more active role in their therapeutic path. Not only patients and clinicians are called to participate in the process of healthcare, but also patients' family and caregivers play an important role. This is even more true in the case of oncological diseases, which have repercussions and consequences not only on the patient but also on people close to him or her (Mohr et al. 1994; Pitceathly and Maguire 2003; Woźniak and Iżycki 2014). Within the iManageCancer platform, the serious game is the app that more effectively promote social wellbeing. Serious games are meant to support the patient in reducing stress, anxiety, and related negative impact of the disease on their lives and social relations and thus to contribute to keep a positive attitude towards the disease and life (Kelley et al. 2017; Sardi et al. 2017). In addition, family resilience is an important factor in the oncological therapeutic path, which is why family members are encouraged to answer the FaRe questionnaire (available on the iPHR), allowing the healthcare professionals to capture any uneasy situations and intervene. The iManageCancer platform mostly encourages a more direct involvement from the patient but also involves families and caregivers, thus promoting an effective alliance among all the actors of the therapeutic path, according to the P5 *participatory* property (Gorini and Pravettoni 2011; Kabat-Zinn 2000).

The iManageCancer project perfectly matches the *psychocognitive* approach suggested by Pravettoni and Gorini (Gorini and Pravettoni 2011; Pravettoni and Gorini 2011); its objective is the patient's empowerment, starting from the belief that patient empowerment in medical care is only possible if based on a multi-level consideration of patients. As a matter of fact, the platform itself promotes a broad consideration of patient health: every feature of the platform has been designed to meet all the need of patients in managing their health as persons and therefore as a set of complex biological systems but also as a subject of emotions, fears, hopes, and needs, who has relationships and lives in a social context. In some cases, the idea behind an application has been to support an all-inclusive wellbeing of patients, with a specific focus on the psychological aspects.

Above all the apps, the serious game aims at helping patients to manage the psychological impact of the diagnosis and consequent treatment. Serious games have been proposed as a strategy to encourage healthy habits and the participation in social life, face disease in a different perspective, and promote illness management (Hoffmann and Wilson 2018; Kelley et al. 2017; Sardi et al. 2017). Serious games can also enhance patient's knowledge through education, reduce feelings of uncertainty, and simultaneously increase confidence in decision-making. From this perspective, serious games will provide also the opportunity to experience skills and coping strategies in facing cancer (Reichlin et al. 2011).

The iPHR also promotes a personalised approach, as it gives patients the chance to fill the previously mentioned questionnaire; this provides clinicians an interactive psychoemotional health assessment tool for the monitoring of psychological and physiological health status of patients.

4 Conclusion

The advances of technology allow today an ever better degree of participation, thanks to the tools of virtual and augmented reality that offer a much more direct interaction between the user and the external environment and a much more all-encompassing experience. Also in terms of prevention, research combined with eHealth can go a long way, exploiting the potential for data collection and interaction with the user of today's tools in conjunction with recent knowledge in systems biology.

Certainly, we can say that iManageCancer is an attempt to put technology at the service of medicine, with the aim of giving patients a device that can increase the involvement in their own care path, and clinicians a set of tools to personalise care processes by the consideration of patient as a whole, from biological factors to quality of life. As we have extensively debated, every constituent aspect of patients as human beings has been taken into account in the design and development of the platform. Thanks to the first tests of usability, the platform has been renewed for the first time, and the pilot study on efficacy will allow us to rethink and implement some of the functions of the platform, in order to always meet the requests of patients and respond more effectively to their concrete needs during the course of care. P5 considers the impact on quality of life as an additional fundamental marker of effectiveness.

References

Cutica, I., Vie, G. M., & Pravettoni, G. (2014). Personalised medicine: The cognitive side of patients. *European Journal of Internal Medicine, 25*(8), 685–688. https://doi.org/10.1016/j.ejim.2014.07.002.

Faccio, F., Renzi, C., Crico, C., Kazantzaki, E., Kondylakis, H., Koumakis, L., … Pravettoni, G. (2018). Development of an eHealth tool for cancer patients: Monitoring psycho-emotional aspects with the Family Resilience (FaRe) questionnaire. *Ecancermedicalscience, 12*, 852. https://doi.org/10.3332/ecancer.2018.852.

Favrod, J., & Khazaal, Y. (2018). *Computers and games for mental health and well-being*. Lausanne: Frontiers Media.

Fleming, P. S., Koletsi, D., Ioannidis, J. P. A., & Pandis, N. (2016). High quality of the evidence for medical and other health-related interventions was uncommon in Cochrane systematic reviews. *Journal of Clinical Epidemiology, 78*, 34–42. https://doi.org/10.1016/j.jclinepi.2016.03.012.

Gorini, A., & Pravettoni, G. (2011). P5 medicine: A plus for a personalized approach to oncology. *Nature Reviews Clinical Oncology, 8*(7), 444. https://doi.org/10.1038/nrclinonc.2010.227-c1.

Gorini, A., Mazzocco, K., Gandini, S., Munzone, E., McVie, G., & Pravettoni, G. (2015). Development and psychometric testing of a breast cancer patient-profiling questionnaire. *Breast Cancer (Dove Medical Press), 7*, 133–146. https://doi.org/10.2147/BCTT.S80014.

Hoffmann, S., & Wilson, S. (2018). The role of serious games in the iManageCancer project. *Ecancermedicalscience, 12*, 850. https://doi.org/10.3332/ecancer.2018.850.

Kabat-Zinn, J. (2000). Participatory medicine. *Journal of the European Academy of Dermatology and Venereology*. https://doi.org/10.1046/j.1468-3083.2000.00062.x.

Kelley, C., Wilcox, L., Ng, W., Schiffer, J., & Hammer, J. (2017). Design features in games for health: Disciplinary and interdisciplinary expert perspectives. *DIS. Designing Interactive Systems (Conference), 2017*, 69–81. https://doi.org/10.1145/3064663.3064721.

Kim, I., Choi, H. J., Ryu, J. M., Lee, S. K., Yu, J. H., Kim, S. W., … Lee, J. E. (2018). A predictive model for high/low risk group according to oncotype DX recurrence score using machine learning. *European Journal of Surgical Oncology*. https://doi.org/10.1016/j.ejso.2018.09.011

Kondylakis, H., Bucur, A., Dong, F., Renzi, C., Manfrinati, A., Graf, N., et al. (2017). iManagecancer: Developing a platform for empowering patients and strengthening self-management in cancer diseases. In *Computer-based medical systems (CBMS), 2017 IEEE 30th international symposium on* (pp. 755–760). Los Alamitos: IEEE.

Mohr, V., Allen, S., & Malin, M. (1994). The psychosocial impact of cancer on older versus younger patients and their families. *Cancer, 74*(S7), 2118–2127.

Nobel, C. (2011). Teaching a 'Lean Startup' strategy. *HBS Working Knowledge*, pp 1–2.

Pitceathly, C., & Maguire, P. (2003). The psychological impact of cancer on patients' partners and other key relatives: A review. *European Journal of Cancer, 39*(11), 1517–1524. https://doi.org/10.1016/S0959-8049(03)00309-5.

Pravettoni, G., & Gorini, A. (2011). A P5 cancer medicine approach: Why personalized medicine cannot ignore psychology. *Journal of Evaluation in Clinical Practice, 17*(4), 594–596. https://doi.org/10.1111/j.1365-2753.2011.01709.x.

Reichlin, L., Mani, N., McArthur, K., Harris, A. M., Rajan, N., & Dacso, C. C. (2011). Assessing the acceptability and usability of an interactive serious game in aiding treatment decisions for patients with localized prostate cancer. *Journal of Medical Internet Research, 13*(1), e4. https://doi.org/10.2196/jmir.1519.

Renzi, C., Riva, S., Masiero, M., & Pravettoni, G. (2016). The choice dilemma in chronic hematological conditions: Why choosing is not only a medical issue? A psycho-cognitive perspective. *Critical Reviews in Oncology/Hematology.* https://doi.org/10.1016/j.critrevonc.2015.12.010.

Sardi, L., Idri, A., & Fernández-Alemán, J. L. (2017). A systematic review of gamification in e-health. *Journal of Biomedical Informatics, 71*, 31–48. https://doi.org/10.1016/J.JBI.2017.05.011.

Schwaber, K., & Beedle, M. (2002). *Agile software development with scrum* (Vol. 1). Upper Saddle River: Prentice Hall.

Woźniak, K., & Iżycki, D. (2014). Cancer: A family at risk. *Przeglad Menopauzalny = Menopause Review, 13*(4), 253–261. https://doi.org/10.5114/pm.2014.45002.

Zhang, X., Deng, Z., Parvinzamir, F., & Dong, F. (2018). MyHealthAvatar lifestyle management support for cancer patients. *Ecancermedicalscience, 12*, 849. https://doi.org/10.3332/ecancer.2018.849.

Part II
The 5 Ps and eHealth

Chapter 3
The Prevention of Chronic Diseases Through eHealth: A Practical Overview

Dario Monzani and Silvia Francesca Maria Pizzoli

1 Introduction

The implementation of effective prevention programs delivered through eHealth technologies is a promising approach to prevent the onset and progression of chronic conditions as P5 underlines. Specifically, eHealth prevention interventions combine the effectiveness of the traditional preventive programs with substantial advantages and functionalities of the new technologies.

Indeed, eHealth prevention interventions allow to target larger segments of population, by giving each individual tailored and real-time feedback (cfr. Chap. 4) about personal risk and behaviors (Baker 2001; Evers 2005; Fotheringham et al. 2000).

Nowadays, chronic diseases are the leading cause of disability and mortality all over the world (World Health Organization 2009, 2017). According to the World Health Organization, chronic diseases are illnesses with a slow progression and prolonged duration; they generally do not resolve spontaneously and could be treated but rarely cured completely (World Health Organization 2017). They could be defined as health conditions lasting 3 months or more that could not be prevented by vaccines or cured by medications (MedicineNet 2016). Time duration and the fact that symptom control is the primary scope of the cure render chronic conditions a relevant issue for patients and for the healthcare system.

All chronic conditions are characterized by four main common qualities (Australian Institute of Health and Welfare 2016). First, they are typified by complex and multiple causalities because their onset and progression are influenced by

D. Monzani (✉) · S. F. M. Pizzoli
Department of Oncology and Hemato-Oncology, University of Milan, Milan, Italy

Applied Research Division for Cognitive and Psychological Science,
European Institute of Oncology (IEO) IRCCS, Milan, Italy
e-mail: dario.monzani@ieo.it; silviafrancescamaria.pizzoli@ieo.it

G. Pravettoni, S. Triberti (eds.), *P5 eHealth: An Agenda for the Health Technologies of the Future*, https://doi.org/10.1007/978-3-030-27994-3_3

several interacting factors, such as genetic, environmental, and behavioral factors. Second, chronic conditions generally start with early developmental phases that are often asymptomatic and then develop slowly. Third, they display a prolonged course of illness that generally flows into other related health complications. Finally, chronic diseases lead to several and serious impairment or disability. Heart disease, cancer, type 2 diabetes, arthritis, Alzheimer' disease, depression, HIV, hypertension, chronic respiratory diseases, and asthma are among the most prototypical example of this kind of health conditions. Chronic respiratory diseases, cardiovascular diseases, cancer, and diabetes are the most widespread chronic conditions worldwide (World Health Organization 2015). Their burden is a common challenge for developing and developed countries; because of their huge health and economic costs, they constitute one of the main challenges for healthcare systems around the world. Together, they account for more than 30 million of deaths of people between the ages 30 and 70 years (World Health Organization 2017). Hundreds of millions of people suffer from chronic respiratory diseases worldwide (World Health Organization 2008a) and diabetes (International Diabetes Federation 2018), while in middle- and low-income countries, the percentage of deaths ascribed to cardiovascular diseases is nearly 30% of the all-cause mortality (World Health Organization 2008b). New cases of worldwide cancer are estimated around 14.1 million of people each year (Cancer Research UK 2018). Globally, most deaths for chronic diseases might be avoided or at least delayed by implementing and delivering effective interventions aimed at preventing or controlling these conditions.

2 Risk Factors for Chronic Diseases

The first necessary step in the effective prevention of each chronic condition is the identification of substantial risk factors for its onset, development, and progression (World Health Organization 2009). Several risk factors for chronic diseases have been described, and they can be classified as non-modifiable and modifiable risk factors. The first ones refer to causes and conditions out of people's control and that could not be changed or treated. Age, gender, ethnicity, genetic, and family history (cfr. Chap. 4) are among the most important and common non-modifiable risk factors for several chronic diseases, such as cardiovascular diseases (Sharkey and Modarai 2018), cancer (Nindrea et al. 2018; World Health Organization 2015), chronic obtrusive respiratory disease (Singanayagam et al. 2013), and type 2 diabetes (Seuring et al. 2015). On the other hand, modifiable risk factors are aspects that could be treated, controlled, and changed and that are, at least at some degree, under subjects' will. They include overweight or obesity, cigarette smoking, physical inactivity, high-cholesterol or lipid levels, and high blood pressure. These modifiable risk factors can be targeted efficiently by implementing effective interventions to promote health, salutogenic lifestyles, and behavioral change. It is also relevant to stress that a bunch of modifiable risk factors are responsible for the onset and progression of several health chronic conditions. For example, cardiovascular diseases, obtrusive respiratory conditions, diabetes, and cancer share the same modifiable risk factors. Specifically, the most deadly modifiable risk factors for these chronic conditions are hypertension (responsible for more than 10% of global deaths each year), tobacco (9%), hypercholesterolemia (6%), sedentariness, and obesity (5%) (World Health Organization 2009).

3 Primary, Secondary, and Tertiary eHealth Prevention

Each eHealth prevention intervention could be adequately described by considering a bunch of conceptual and practical aspects that were commonly used to elucidate differences among traditional preventive efforts. The first distinction refers to primary, secondary, and tertiary prevention (Institute for Work and Health 2018). Specifically, primary prevention is aimed at preventing diseases and medical conditions before they occur. Primary preventive efforts try to avoid the exposures to environmental risk, inform and educate people about unsafe and healthy habits, and target modifiable risk factors, such as unsafe behaviors or unhealthy habits, through lifestyle modification. For example, several mHealth interventions have been implemented to promote healthy sun-related behaviors and attitudes to prevent skin cancer (for a review, see Finch et al. 2016). These interventions were primarily informative and educational about the risk of unprotected exposure to the UV radiation and were delivered through daily text messages, e-mails, and written reminders asking people to apply sunscreen protection. Secondary preventive efforts are aimed at reducing the impact of disease or medical conditions through their early detection and treatment in order to mitigate their impact and slowdown progression. eHealth secondary prevention interventions especially focus on monitoring symptomatology and promoting screening behavior. Prototypical examples of eHealth secondary prevention are mobile applications aimed at facilitating early detection of melanoma in people at high risk for developing melanoma by promoting annual total body skin exams and instructing about the skin self-examination (for a review, see Wu et al. (2016)). Specifically, the SkinVision mHealth, an integrated risk assessment algorithm for melanocytic lesions and melanoma detection, evaluates picture taken with the smartphone camera and then gives user useful information about each lesion and its associated risk for developing skin cancer (Thissen et al. 2017; Udrea and Lupu 2014). From this point of view, this mobile app could be a useful eHealth secondary prevention effort to detect melanoma in early stages, mitigate its possible progression, and then potentially reduce rates of mortality for skin cancer. Finally, tertiary prevention interventions focus especially on patients' self-management abilities, efficient proactive strategies, and lifestyle modification to prevent recurrence, progression, and long-term severe outcomes of the disease. The specific aim of this kind of eHealth intervention is to soften the impact of an ongoing chronic disease or medical conditions. Tertiary prevention intervention through mobile technologies was recently implemented to promote self-management abilities, self-care, and glycemic control in patients with type 2 diabetes (for a review, see Wu et al. (2018)). These mobile apps permit patients to monitor automatically and real-time the glucose level through a wireless glucometer, store this information in the smartphone, and receive personalized information with remainders, motivational message, and indication about lifestyle modifications.

4 Population-Based vs. Individual-Based eHealth Prevention

Alongside classification among primary, secondary, and tertiary prevention, eHealth prevention intervention could be categorized by referring to the specific target population of their preventive effort. Specifically, the epidemiologist Geoffrey Rose proposed a relevant distinction among different strategies for the prevention of chronic conditions and health problems. He stated that preventive efforts could be efficiently implemented by adopting one of the two main approaches or strategies to prevention: the population-based and the individual high-risk approaches (Rose 1995). The first one targets the entire population with health promotion actions and activities that prevent disease and negative outcomes through the implementation of policies and interventions aimed at promoting population-based behavioral change and healthy lifestyle and influencing the physical, social, and economic environment. Through the adoption of new technologies, innovative eHealth prevention interventions could be potentiality delivered to a wider audience than the one reached with traditional approaches for the prevention of chronic diseases. One example of a population-based mHealth preventive strategy is the Stroke Riskometer app for the primary prevention (Feigin et al. 2015, 2017; Parmar et al. 2015). This mobile application informs the general population about individual and overall risk for stroke, educates people about warning signs of stroke, and empowers them with effective strategies to reduce their cardiovascular risk by providing evidence-based and internationally recognized guidelines about pharmacological treatment and behavioral change.

Conversely, in accordance with the P5 approach, the individual high-risk approach aimed at firstly identifying individuals with high risk for developing diseases or negative outcomes and then targeting this specific population with ad hoc preventive interventions. This kind of prevention strategies focuses especially on individuals with high level of known risk factor for chronic diseases or people that show premorbid signs prior to the onset of illness. Subsequently, personalized health education, health promotion, and behavioral change interventions are delivered to promote healthy lifestyles and reduce risk factors and premorbidity. The adoption of new technologies has the potentiality of boosting the implementation of personalized interventions in medicine (Cutica et al. 2014; Renzi et al. 2016), because they offer unique opportunities to personalize contents and stimuli (Pizzoli et al. 2019). For example, innovative technologies obtain a clear and real-time picture of each individual by taking into account individual risk factor, behaviors, abilities, and needs and then tailor preventive efforts to this specific individual and disease profile (Vergani et al. 2019). One example of an innovative eHealth prevention intervention is the Consumer Navigation of Electronic Cardiovascular Tool (CONNECT; Coorey et al. 2017; Redfern et al. 2014). It is a web application, accessible via a mobile device or computer, delivering a multicomponent and personalized eHealth prevention effort to empower people with moderate-to-high cardiovascular risk in opting for or increasing treatment adherence and healthy lifestyle modifications. CONNECT enables the real-time calculation of individual risk score for cardiovascular diseases. Other core features of this eHealth individual high-risk intervention are tracking of actual behaviors, interactive educational resources about risks and benefits of lifestyle, and delivering of tailored healthy habit recommendations and motivational messages for effective behavioral changes.

5 eHealth Behavioral Change Interventions

Behavioral change techniques and personalized motivational factors for lifestyle modification are among the most common core features of several eHealth interventions to prevent the onset and progression of illnesses. Specifically, the most innovative and promising approaches deliver traditional, theoretical, and evidence-based behavioral change interventions by means of new and digital technologies, such as mobile applications, websites, text messages, and serious games. For what concern behavioral change intervention, starting from the 1950s, several theories and models of behavioral change have been proposed to effectively target health-compromising habits responsible for the onset and progression of acute and chronic diseases. The Health Belief Model (Rosenstock 1974), the Social Cognitive Theory (Bandura 1977), the Transtheoretical Model (Prochaska and Diclemente 1983; Prochaska and Velicer 1997), and the Health Action Process Approach (Schwarzer 1992, 2008; Schwarzer et al. 2011) are the most known clinically and empirically grounded theories of behavioral change. Meta-analytical results demonstrated the superiority, in comparison with usual primary health care, of theoretically based health behavioral change interventions in promoting healthier lifestyle in terms of reduced intake of calories and saturated fats, improvement in intensity and frequency of physical activity, and smoking cessation (Bully et al. 2015). Each model has its specificity in promoting lifestyle modifications (for a brief overview, see Stroebe (2011)). Even if there are radical theoretical and conceptual differences among these models, all of them stress the role of personal control and self-efficacy belief in promoting lifestyle modifications. Specifically, as the P5 approach highlights, they suggest that individuals are more likely to change unhealthy behaviors and to maintain lifestyle modification over time when they perceive themselves as able to effectively succeed in these tasks (Bandura 1977, 1982). For example, people are more likely to quit smoking when they have strong beliefs about their ability to abstain from smoking and maintain abstinence (Gwaltney et al. 2013). Furthermore, self-efficacy beliefs seem to shape the relationship between perceived health satisfaction and illness severity in cardiovascular diseases (Greco et al. 2015; Steca et al. 2013, 2015). As we will deepen in the next section, eHealth interventions have been developed by taking advantage of the technical capabilities of web-based and mobile technologies to track real-time behavioral and health information, involve the healthcare providers, leverage peer and social influence, and increase the accessibility of health information to deliver more effective preventive interventions (Klasnja and Pratt 2012). These technical features are especially useful for the promotion of people's self-efficacy, one of the main core features of both traditional and eHealth preventive interventions, because they permit the real-time monitoring of actual behaviors and then deliver personalized vicarious experience, modeling, and tailored feedbacks. Other determinants of intention to change and actual lifestyle modification have been proposed in the main behavioral change theories. Among these determinants, the most relevant are perceived risk or vulnerability, attitude toward unhealthy and healthy behaviors, and outcome expectancy (Stroebe 2011). Starting from this theoretical knowledge and empirical evidence, several eHealth interventions have approached the prevention of chronic diseases by taking advantage of technical solutions introduced by new media. These eHealth interventions have the qualities of engaging users deeply, permitting an easy integration between usual care and self-management practices, obtaining real-time and online monitoring of clinical outcomes and behaviors, and personalizing feedback and motivational messages to users (Kebede et al. 2017).

Even if some preventive interventions apply theoretical knowledge on behavioral change, two recent meta-analyses on the use of lifestyle modification in web-based and mobile interventions for self-management respectively of asthma (Al-Durra et al. 2015) and type 2 diabetes (Van Vugt et al. 2013) highlighted that a considerable proportion of eHealth preventive efforts does not adopt any documented and empirical-based behavioral change theories. The remaining eHealth interventions adopt the Health Belief Model (Rosenstock 1974), the Transtheoretical Model (Prochaska and Diclemente 1983; Prochaska and Velicer 1997), and the Self-Efficacy and Social-Cognitive Model (Bandura 1977, 1982), alongside with gamification and tailored communication, to promote self-management, self-care, and healthy habits in this kind of patients.

Upon reviewing the literature on mHealth behavioral interventions to counteract physical inactivity and sedentary habits, Direito et al. (2017) highlighted that there is a strong heterogeneity in the terminology used to describe behavioral change interventions. Specifically, in detailing their interventions, developers are more likely to refer to specific core features and strategies rather than reporting actual behavioral change theories and models. Specifically, the vast majority of interventions adopted goal setting, alongside with self-monitoring, social support, feedbacks, and educational components, to foster moderate-to-vigorous physical activity. This kind of techniques implicates the development of a detailed action plan to motivate and orient people toward a meaningful goal (Bryan and Locke 1967; Latham and Locke 2009; Locke and Latham 2006). Goal setting involves the development of an action plan designed to motivate and guide people in goal pursuit. Thus, individuals are educated to establish clear objective about behavioral change, instructed on how to efficiently pursue them, and constantly motivated to reach these specific health-related goals. The importance of establishing clear and detailed objectives for effective behavioral change has been acknowledged by a few eHealth preventive programs that have implemented the SMART criteria. Specifically, SMART goals – which stands for "Specific, Measurable, Achievable, Relevant, and Time Bound" – are the best type of goals to be set (Macleod 2013; Moskowitz and Halvorson 2009). This technique has been implemented in the strengthening and stretching (mySARAH; Srikesavan et al. 2018), an online tertiary preventive effort for people suffering from rheumatoid arthritis of the hand. This web-based program includes educational videos about upper limb mobility exercise and strength exercise for hands. Adherence to the exercise plan is fostered with behavioral support strategies of self-monitoring, goal setting, SMART goals, and action planning. Specifically, patients are asked to set SMART goals about exercise, plan their workout schedule, and constantly review their SMART goals on the basis of actual behaviors and performance.

Overall, in most cases, there is still a lack of evidence-based and solid theoretical foundations of eHealth prevention interventions. However, regardless of the specific behavioral change model being adopted, web-based behavioral change interventions have been demonstrated to be more effective than traditional ones in increasing knowledge about nutrition and physical exercise and people's awareness about health risk factors and individual risk and in promoting subsequent lifestyle modification in terms of being more active and having an healthy diet (Wantland et al. 2004). For example, wearable devices, such activity and sleep trackers and blood pressure and heart monitors, bring new possibilities in delivering effective and tailored behavioral change interventions to increase the frequency and intensity of physical exercise. Results of a recent meta-analysis showed that behavioral change interventions comprising both wearable devices and mobile applications are effective in promoting physical activity, measured through objective measure and daily step count, in the general population (Gal et al. 2018).

To sum up, while several eHealth preventive programs have been developed without referring to a specific theory of behavioral change, the adoption of a solid theoretical foundation is a necessary and preliminary step in the development of this kind of interventions. The selection of the specific behavioral change theory or technique to be implemented in eHealth preventive program aimed at promoting lifestyle modification should be facilitated by considering the classification proposed by Michie and colleagues (Michie et al. 2011, 2013). Specifically, upon reviewing the literature on traditional health behavioral change, they developed an extensive and useful taxonomy of 93 hierarchically clustered techniques that could be used to implement lifestyle modification interventions through eHealth modalities. As stated by Van Vugt et al. (2013), the selection of the specific technology of an eHealth intervention is secondary and should follow the decision about the specific behavioral change theory or strategy to be implemented. All these steps must be guided by a critical evaluation of theories, empirical evidence, contextual background, and specific nature of the behavior to be targeted.

6 Strategies of eHealth Prevention

The classification proposed by Michie and colleagues highlighted a huge heterogeneity in strategies being implemented in traditional intervention programs aimed at promoting preventive habits and lifestyle modifications. Specifically, through a consensus exercise involving more than 50 experts in implementing and delivering lifestyle modification interventions, they developed a list of 93 strategies to promote behavioral change. These methods have been subsequently clustered into high-order classes of (1) reinforcement (e.g., punishment, response cost, chaining), (2) reward and threat (e.g., social and self-reward), (3) repetition and substitution (e.g., Behavioral substitution, habit formation, and reversal), (4) antecedents (e.g., restructuring the social and physical environment), (5) associative learning (e.g., exposure, classical conditioning, and prompt cues), (6) covert learning (e.g., vicarious reinforcement and convert conditioning), (7) consequences (e.g., salience of consequences, health and emotional consequences), (8) feedback and monitoring (e.g., feedback on behavior, biofeedback, and self-monitoring of behavior), (9) goals and planning (e.g., action planning including implementation intention and goal setting), (10) social support (e.g., practical and emotional support), (11) comparison of behavior (e.g., modeling of behavior and social comparison, (12) self-belief (e.g., self-task, focus on past success, and verbal persuasion to boost self-efficacy), (13) comparison of outcomes (e.g., persuasive argument, pros, and cons), (14) identity (e.g., self-affirmation and cognitive dissonance), (15) shaping knowledge (e.g., reattribution and instructions on how to perform a behavior), and (16) regulation (e.g., regulate negative emotions, pharmacological support, and conserving mental resources) (for a review, see Michie et al. (2011, 2013)).

The vast majority of these overarching strategies have been transferred and adapted to deliver eHealth prevention and behavioral change intervention while taking advantage of the technical capabilities of the World Wide Web, personal computers, smartphones and mobile apps, and wearable devices. In 2012, Klasnja and Pratt (2012) developed a concise taxonomy of strategies that have been generally used in mobile-based healthcare interventions. Specifically, four of these core strategies might be used to describe each eHealth prevention effort: (1) promoting health information and awareness, (2) tracking behavioral and health information, (3) leveraging social influence, and (4) utilizing entertainment and gamification. Generally, effective eHealth preventive efforts rely on a peculiar combination of two or more of these strategies.

One of the core components of most eHealth interventions (and also of the P5 approach) is educational and information feature aimed at promoting awareness and knowledge about health and risk factor for the onset and progression of chronic diseases and reminding and motivating users or patients to promote their self-management abilities, treatment adherence, and behavioral change. New media technologies permit to deliver health information to a wider audience than the one possible reached by traditional prevention program. Web-based and interactive educational efforts that allow users to navigate through online information on their own are effective in increasing self-management abilities and self-care habits for the secondary and tertiary prevention of illnesses and medical conditions (Fredericks et al. 2015; Webb et al. 2010). This kind of interventions is especially useful for the prevention of chronic diseases because it allows people to access autonomously relevant health information and decide the type and amount of data they are willing to consult. For example, HeartCare is an intervention dealing with the secondary and tertiary prevention of chronic cardiac diseases. It is a web-based tool aimed at improving self-care and adherence to treatment by allowing patients to access useful information on their disease, medication, and behavioral recommendations, in terms of diet and physical activity (Brennan et al. 2001, 2010). This kind of web-based educational intervention is more cost-effective than the traditional ones in delivering evidence-based and specialized health information to acute and chronic patients (Brennan et al. 2010; Côté et al. 2011; Martorella et al. 2012; Runge et al. 2006). Indeed, educational eHealth interventions strongly rely on the involvement and engagement of people that are requested to actively search and autonomously consult information about their health and behaviors.

On the contrary, other technologies, such as text messages and notifications from mobile apps, permit to deliver health information, prompts, and reminders to people that receive them without any active searching or commitment and permit to provide information at the right time (e.g., at dinner time when patients should take medications). Text messages and notifications could be used as (1) educational content, (2) prompts to remind patients to take their medications, and (3) tips to motivate them to behavioral change. For example, daily phone text messages have been used to promote self-care and adherence to treatment in people suffering from chronic respiratory diseases (Strandbygaard et al. 2010). General educational messages are used to inform users or patients about their health condition, symptomatology, possible preventive efforts, and lifestyle modification that could counteract the onset or progression of medical conditions (Beratarrechea et al. 2017; Orr and King 2015). The adoption of eHealth modalities allows the easy implementation of tailored or personalized communication that, compared to generic information, is more effective in promoting lifestyle modification and screening behaviors (Ovbiagele et al. 2015). Moreover, text messages and notifications might be used as prompts to remind users and patients to take medications or to engage in a specific behavior. This is particularly useful in behavioral change interventions to increase users' perseverance and consistency in performing preventive and health-promoting actions that they are very likely to forget to do. Finally, personalized education and informative contents could be also used as tips or advices to motivate users to change their unhealthy behaviors or be adherent to treatment by teaching them effective strategies on how to counteract to obstacles and difficulties interfering with adherence and behavioral change (Gerber et al. 2009).

Nowadays, mobile applications and new wearable devices allow the constant and automated monitoring of users' behaviors and clinical conditions, in accordance with the P5 approach. The key core of many eHealth prevention interventions takes advantage from the possibility to easily track physiological parameters, health-related behaviors, and psychological states. Patients could track and record all these data by (1) using automated sensors and (2) actively logging behaviors, health information, and medication. Self-monitoring is a viable strategy to prevent illness and foster healthy behavioral change by promoting patients' awareness about their own health and health-related behaviors, motivating users in treatment adherence and behavioral change recommendations, and promoting frequency of healthy habits (Consolvo et al. 2008; Gasser et al. 2006; Nelson 1977; Ness et al. 2007). Furthermore, constant and recorded information on physiological parameters allow and facilitate the participation and inclusion of informal caregivers and healthcare providers in patients' self-management process. This feature is especially relevant for the secondary and tertiary prevention because people suffering from chronic diseases are generally required to monitor their symptomatology, adhere to complex treatment, and maintain healthy habits. A bunch of eHealth intervention monitor patients' conditions and alert healthcare providers or informal caregivers where severe clinical outcome has been detected. For example, a complex system of wearable devices consisting of a high blood pressure bracelet, ECG sensor, and accelerometers permits patients with chronic heart failure or heart diseases to automatically record their health status (Rubel et al. 2004, 2005; Villalba Mora et al. 2006, 2009). Informal caregivers and the healthcare team are automatically contacted if necessary. As mentioned above, accelerometer, activity and sleep trackers, blood and heart rate sensors, and step counter integrated in many smartphones are useful wearable devices that foster the possibilities of new eHealth preventive efforts to increase behavioral change, especially in terms of increasing physical exercise (Gal et al. 2018). Self-monitoring is also an effective way to promote weight management for the prevention of obesity and overweight problems in adult populations (Burke et al. 2011; Madigan et al. 2015; Zheng et al. 2015). As highlighted by a recent meta-analysis by Ho et al. (2018), many eHealth programs delivered web-based self-monitoring to prevent obesity during adolescence as well. All these assessed studies employed logging of behaviors and health information that, differently from automated tracking of personal information through wearable devices, requires users to provide and record all the relevant health-related data. Specifically, adolescents are asked to daily log information about their diet, physical activity, and weight. Results suggested that daily self-monitoring, supported by goal setting and face-to-face counseling, is effective in reducing adolescents' body mass index.

Besides being positive influenced by individual engagement and active effort, the effective health promotion, lifestyle modifications, and preventive interventions are leveraged by a supportive social environment for patients and users. Specifically, emotional and instrumental social support from partners, relatives, and friends may facilitate self-care, behavioral change, and adherence to treatment in healthy people and patients with chronic diseases (Finlay et al. 2018; Holt-Lunstad 2018; Lange et al. 2018; Tregarthen et al. 2015; Uchino et al. 2018). By recognizing the pivotal role of social influence and support for the effectiveness of each preventive effort, several traditional and eHealth interventions have included specific features aimed at leveraging social influence to promote self-management skills, screening behaviors, lifestyle modifications, and treatment adherence. There are three main strategies that have been implemented within eHealth preventive programs to take advantage of social influence for health promotion by leveraging (1) social support from family and friends (cfr. Chap. 4), (2) peer-to-peer influence, and (3) vicarious experience and peer modeling.

The first strategy might be especially useful for people facing strong difficulties in changing their unhealthy habits or maintaining an adequate self-care. In this case, close relatives and friends may support and motivate those people in accomplishing their health-related goals and improving their self-management skills. An eHealth preventive program aimed at helping people quit smoking by leveraging social support from a support person nominated by the quitter is an example of this category (Obermayer et al. 2004). Specifically, this web-based intervention allows the support person to constantly monitor the progress of the quitter and then send the abstinence smoker motivational and supporting text messages. The second strategy aims at leveraging social influence by allowing interaction among people working on the same health-related task. This might be especially useful either for sharing how-to practices, reassurance, encouragement, and information or motivating people through competition. Peer-to-peer social support allows sharing instrumental information on strategies and practical instructions on how to effectively deal with self-care practices, behavioral change, and adherence to treatment and also foster discussions about feelings and emotions or share encouragement, reflection, and reassurance among users. For example, a bunch of eHealth intervention for the promotion of physical activity have implemented peer-to-peer discussion boards, buddy systems (i.e., two or more people are able to monitor and help each other), live chats, and forums to allow people to motivate each other and share their feelings and thoughts about physical exercise (Webb et al. 2010). On the contrary, other eHealth interventions have adopted peer-to-peer competition to foster motivation in changing unhealthy lifestyles. For example, Mobile Lifestyle Coach app used competition among users to boost their levels of physical activity and their healthy nutritional habits (Gasser et al. 2006). As this mobile app employed also gamification, users were assigned into teams that compete one against the other. The winning team is the one that obtains the higher individual and cumulative scores of healthy habits measured as progress toward daily goals of balanced diet and physical activity. Peer-to-peer influence and social support from family might be powerful strategies to enhance people's self-efficacy in following preventive programs and recommendations for behavioral change. In fact, as clearly stated by Bandura (1977, 1982), people's belief about their ability to succeed in a specific task can be developed by four main sources of influence: (1) mastery or enactive experience (success increases perceived self-efficacy and failure reduces it); (2) vicarious experience or modeling (when people observe someone succeeding in a task, their self-efficacy generally increases); (3) verbal and social persuasion (motivational feedback and direct encouragement from other people might foster individual self-efficacy); and

(4) physiological factors (perception and belief about sign of distress, such as negative emotion, fatigue, and pain, may alter self-efficacy). eHealth providing peer-to-peer influence and social support from family and friends might be especially helpful for people dealing with complex health-related task such as lifestyle modification because these strategies allow people to receive verbal persuasion about their ability to alter given tasks and thus catalyze greater effort. Also the third and last strategy of leveraging social influence through vicarious experience and modeling may be relevant to foster people self-efficacy. Specifically, this approach relies on the power of peer-to-peer exchange of useful information about tips and effective strategies to effectively deal with behavioral change and overcome health-related difficulties. Successful peers are thus competent and proficient models that disseminate effective skills and schemes for managing task demands that consequently raise perceived efficacy. For example, Schweier et al. (2014) have developed a web-based peer-modeling intervention to promote healthy lifestyle changes and self-management ability in German patients with cardiovascular diseases and chronic back pain. Their open access and no-cost website provides more than 1000 texts, audios, and videos of people with coronary heart disease and chronic back pain reporting how they had efficiently modified their unhealthy behaviors focusing on obstacles and their successful strategies in maintaining healthy habits.

Overall, eHealth behavioral change and preventive interventions must face the main challenge of motivating people to act appropriately and to maintain lifestyle modifications over time. It is often hard to motivate healthy but physical inactive people in changing their unhealthy habits. Furthermore, most people are very likely to adhere to an eHealth preventive program only for a short time. However, it is possible to take advantage of the motivational capacity of entertainment content, gamification, and games to keep users engaged (Craig Lefebvre et al. 2010; Gal et al. 2018; Graffigna et al. 2014; McCallum 2012; Sardi et al. 2017). As the P5 approach suggests, the use of entertainment content and gamification has been adopted as one of the four core strategies of many eHealth prevention interventions.

One prototypical example of the power of gamification to motivate people to be more physically active is Pokémon GO, a commercial mobile-augmented reality game that has been proved effective in fostering physical activity in young and inactive people (Althoff et al. 2016; Gabbiadini et al. 2018; Howe et al. 2016). Similarly, gamification has been implemented in REACH for Success, an innovative mHealth prevention and early intervention program targeting anxious symptomatology in youth (Stoll et al. 2017). Specifically, this mobile app relies on gamification to increase people's engagement and adoption of effective self-management strategies for managing stress and anxiety-provoking situations. An animated avatar, shaped like a blob, delivers personalized motivational messages and interacts with the user. This avatar is designed following the *Proteus effect* positing that animated representation that rewards people for being successful in a task increased motivation to perform such activity (Yee and Bailenson 2007). When users complete daily homework delivered by REACH, they can tap on the blob and see it performing some leveled tricks.

7 Conclusion

This chapter briefly introduced the eHealth approach to the primary, secondary, and tertiary prevention of chronic diseases. Compared to traditional interventions, eHealth prevention programs can offer several additional benefits. Specifically, this kind of interventions takes advantage from the huge functionalities of new technologies that allow people to access easily and briefly health information and educational content, to constantly monitor their health status and behavior, and also to receive real-time and personalized feedbacks about the appropriateness of their actions and about their physiological parameters. Moreover, new media allow an easy and online communication of patients with their caregivers and their peers as well. All these features might be especially relevant in facilitating and motivating people to adopt and maintain healthy lifestyles and subsequently prevent the onset or progression of several chronic conditions. Finally, thanks to the possibility of employing gamification, eHealth interventions might better motivate people to follow preventive and lifestyle modification programs over a long time. For all these reasons, eHealth preventive interventions are promising ways to approach efficiently the primary, secondary, and tertiary prevention of chronic diseases.

Acknowledgment Silvia Francesca Maria Pizzoli is a PhD student within the European School of Molecular Medicine (SEMM).

References

Al-Durra, M., Torio, M. B., & Cafazzo, J. A. (2015). The use of behavior change theory in internet-based asthma self-management interventions: A systematic review. *Journal of Medical Internet Research, 17*(4), e89. https://doi.org/10.2196/jmir.4110.

Althoff, T., White, R. W., & Horvitz, E. (2016). Influence of pokémon go on physical activity: Study and implications. *Journal of Medical Internet Research, 18*(12), 1–14. https://doi.org/10.2196/jmir.6759.

Australian Institute of Health and Welfare. (2016). *Chronic diseases*. Australian Institute of Health and Welfare. Retrieved October 16, 2018, from https://www.aihw.gov.au/reports-data/health-conditions-disability-deaths/chronic-disease/about.

Baker, D. (2001). Patient-centered healthcare: The role of the internet. *Disease Management and Health Outcomes, 9*, 411. https://doi.org/10.2165/00115677-200109080-00001.

Bandura, A. (1977). Self-efficacy: Toward a unifying theory of behavioral change. *Psychological Review, 84*(2), 191–215. https://doi.org/10.1037/0033-295X.84.2.191.

Bandura, A. (1982). Self-efficacy mechanism in human agency. *American Psychologist, 37*, 122. https://doi.org/10.1037/0003-066X.37.2.122.

Beratarrechea, A., Moyano, D., Irazola, V., & Rubinstein, A. (2017). mHealth interventions to counter noncommunicable diseases in developing countries. *Cardiology Clinics, 35*(1), 13–30. https://doi.org/10.1016/j.ccl.2016.08.009.

Brennan, P. F., Casper, G. R., Burke, L. J., Johnson, K. A., Brown, R., Valdez, R. S., … Sturgeon, B. (2010). Technology-enhanced practice for patients with chronic cardiac disease: Home implementation and evaluation. *Heart and Lung: Journal of Acute and Critical Care, 39*(6), S34–S46. https://doi.org/10.1016/j.hrtlng.2010.09.003.

Brennan, P. F., Moore, S. M., Bjornsdottir, G., Jones, J., Visovsky, C., & Rogers, M. (2001). HeartCare: An internet-based information and support system for patient home recovery after coronary artery bypass graft (CABG) surgery. *Journal of Advanced Nursing, 35*(5), 699–708. https://doi.org/10.1046/j.1365-2648.2001.01902.x.

Bryan, J. F., & Locke, E. a. (1967). Goal setting as a means of increasing motivation. *The Journal of Applied Psychology, 51*(3), 274–277. https://doi.org/10.1037/h0024566.

Bully, P., Sánchez, Á., Zabaleta-del-Olmo, E., Pombo, H., & Grandes, G. (2015). Evidence from interventions based on theoretical models for lifestyle modification (physical activity, diet, alcohol and tobacco use) in primary care settings: A systematic review. *Preventive Medicine, 76*(S), S76–S93. https://doi.org/10.1016/j.ypmed.2014.12.020.

Burke, L. E., Wang, J., & Sevick, M. A. (2011). Self-monitoring in weight loss: A systematic review of the literature. *Journal of the American Dietetic Association, 111*(1), 92–102. https://doi.org/10.1016/J.JADA.2010.10.008.

Cancer Research UK. (2018). *Worldwide cancer statistics*. Cancer Research UK. Retrieved October 16, 2018, from https://www.cancerresearchuk.org/health-professional/cancer-statistics/worldwide-cancer

Consolvo, S., Klasnja, P., McDonald, D. W., Avrahami, D., Froehlich, J., LeGrand, L., … Landay, J. A. (2008). Flowers or a robot army?: Encouraging awareness & activity with personal, mobile displays. In: *Proceedings of the 10th international conference on ubiquitous computing (UbiComp '08)*, (pp. 54–63). https://doi.org/10.1145/1409635.1409644.

Coorey, G. M., Neubeck, L., Usherwood, T., Peiris, D., Parker, S., Lau, A. Y. S., … Redfern, J. (2017). Implementation of a consumer-focused eHealth intervention for people with moderate-to-high cardiovascular disease risk: Protocol for a mixed-methods process evaluation. *BMJ Open, 7*(1), e014353. https://doi.org/10.1136/bmjopen-2016-014353.

Côté, J., Ramirez-Garcia, P., Rouleau, G., Saulnier, D., Guéhéneuc, Y. G., Hernandez, A., & Godin, G. (2011). A nursing virtual intervention: Real-time support for managing antiretroviral therapy. *CIN – Computers Informatics Nursing, 29*(1), 43–51. https://doi.org/10.1097/NCN.0b013e3181f9dc02.

Craig Lefebvre, R., Tada, Y., Hilfiker, S. W., & Baur, C. (2010). The assessment of user engagement with eHealth content: The eHealth engagement scale. *Journal of Computer-Mediated Communication, 15*(4), 666–681. https://doi.org/10.1111/j.1083-6101.2009.01514.x.

Cutica, I., Vie, G. M., & Pravettoni, G. (2014). Personalised medicine: The cognitive side of patients. *European Journal of Internal Medicine, 25*(8), 685–688. https://doi.org/10.1016/j.ejim.2014.07.002.

Direito, A., Carraça, E., Rawstorn, J., Whittaker, R., & Maddison, R. (2017). mHealth technologies to influence physical activity and sedentary behaviors: Behavior change techniques, systematic review and meta-analysis of randomized controlled trials. *Annals of Behavioral Medicine, 51*, 226. https://doi.org/10.1007/s12160-016-9846-0.

Evers, K. (2005). eHealth promotion: The use of the internet for health promotion. *American Journal of Health Promotion, 20*, iii.

Feigin, V. L., Krishnamurthi, R., Bhattacharjee, R., Parmar, P., Theadom, A., Hussein, T., … Moran, A. E. (2015). New strategy to reduce the global burden of stroke. *Stroke, 46*(6), 1740–1747. https://doi.org/10.1161/STROKEAHA.115.008222.

Feigin, V. L., Norrving, B., & Mensah, G. A. (2017). Primary prevention of cardiovascular disease through population-wide motivational strategies: Insights from using smartphones in stroke prevention. *BMJ Global Health, 2*(2), e000306. https://doi.org/10.1136/bmjgh-2017-000306.

Finch, L., Janda, M., Loescher, L. J., & Hacker, E. (2016). Can skin cancer prevention be improved through mobile technology interventions? A systematic review. *Preventive Medicine, 90*, 121. https://doi.org/10.1016/j.ypmed.2016.06.037.

Finlay, K. A., Peacock, S., & Elander, J. (2018). Developing successful social support: An interpretative phenomenological analysis of mechanisms and processes in a chronic pain support group. *Psychology & Health, 33*(7), 846–871. https://doi.org/10.1080/08870446.2017.1421188.

Fotheringham, M. J., Owies, D., Leslie, E., & Owen, N. (2000). Interactive health communication in preventive medicine: Internet-based strategies in teaching and research. *American Journal of Preventive Medicine, 19*(2), 113–120. https://doi.org/10.1016/S0749-3797(00)00188-4.

Fredericks, S., Martorella, G., & Catallo, C. (2015). A systematic review of web-based educational interventions. *Clinical Nursing Research, 24*(1), 91–113. https://doi.org/10.1177/1054773814522829.

Gabbiadini, A., Sagioglou, C., & Greitemeyer, T. (2018). Does Pokémon go lead to a more physically active life style? *Computers in Human Behavior, 84*, 258. https://doi.org/10.1016/j.chb.2018.03.005.

Gal, R., May, A. M., van Overmeeren, E. J., Simons, M., & Monninkhof, E. M. (2018). The effect of physical activity interventions comprising wearables and smartphone applications on physical activity: a systematic review and meta-analysis. *Sports Medicine – Open, 4*(1), 42. https://doi.org/10.1186/s40798-018-0157-9.

Gasser, R., Brodbeck, D., Degen, M., Luthiger, J., Wyss, R., & Reichlin, S. (2006). *Persuasiveness of a Mobile lifestyle coaching application using social facilitation* (pp. 27–38). Berlin/Heidelberg: Springer. https://doi.org/10.1007/11755494_5.

Gerber, B. S., Stolley, M. R., Thompson, A. L., Sharp, L. K., & Fitzgibbon, M. L. (2009). Mobile phone text messaging to promote healthy behaviors and weight loss maintenance: A feasibility study. *Health Informatics Journal, 15*(1), 17–25. https://doi.org/10.1177/1460458208099865.

Graffigna, G., Barello, S., Triberti, S., Wiederhold, B. K., Bosio, A. C., & Riva, G. (2014). Enabling eHealth as a pathway for patient engagement: a toolkit for medical practice. *Studies in Health Technology and Informatics, 199*, 13–21.

Greco, A., Steca, P., Pozzi, R., Monzani, D., Malfatto, G., & Parati, G. (2015). The influence of illness severity on health satisfaction in patients with cardiovascular disease: The mediating role of illness perception and self-efficacy beliefs. *Behavioral Medicine, 41*(1), 9–17.

Gwaltney, C. J., Metrik, J., Shiffman, S., & Manuscript, A. (2013). Self-efficacy and smoking cessation: A meta-analysis. *Psychology of Addictive Behaviors, 23*(1), 1729–1737. https://doi.org/10.1037/a0013529.Self-Efficacy.

Ho, T. J. H., Lee, C. C. S., Wong, S. N., & Lau, Y. (2018). Internet-based self-monitoring interventions for overweight and obese adolescents: A systematic review and meta-analysis. *International Journal of Medical Informatics, 120*(September), 20–30. https://doi.org/10.1016/j.ijmedinf.2018.09.019.

Holt-Lunstad, J. (2018). Why social relationships are important for physical health: A systems approach to understanding and modifying risk and protection. *Annual Review of Psychology, 69*, 437. https://doi.org/10.1146/annurev-psych-122216-011902.

Howe, K. B., Suharlim, C., Ueda, P., Howe, D., Kawachi, I., & Rimm, E. B. (2016). Gotta catch'em all! Pokémon GO and physical activity among young adults: Difference in differences study. *BMJ (Online), 355*, 1–4. https://doi.org/10.1136/bmj.i6270.

Institute for Work & Health. (2018). *Primary, secondary and tertiary prevention*. Institute for Work and Health. Retrieved October 16, 2018, from https://www.iwh.on.ca/what-researchers-mean-by/primary-secondary-and-tertiary-prevention

International Diabetes Federation. (2018). *IDF diabetes atlas – 2017 Atlas*. Retrieved October 16, 2018, from http://diabetesatlas.org/resources/2017-atlas.html

Kebede, M., Christianson, L., Khan, Z., Heise, T. L., & Pischke, C. R. (2017). Effectiveness of behavioral change techniques employed in eHealth interventions designed to improve glycemic control in persons with poorly controlled type 2 diabetes: a systematic review and meta-analysis protocol. *Systematic Reviews, 6*(1), 211. https://doi.org/10.1186/s13643-017-0609-1.

Klasnja, P., & Pratt, W. (2012). Healthcare in the pocket: Mapping the space of mobile-phone health interventions. *Journal of Biomedical Informatics, 45*, 184. https://doi.org/10.1016/j.jbi.2011.08.017.

Lange, D., Corbett, J., Knoll, N., Schwarzer, R., & Lippke, S. (2018). Fruit and vegetable intake: The interplay of planning, social support, and sex. *International Journal of Behavioral Medicine, 25*(4), 421–430. https://doi.org/10.1007/s12529-018-9718-z.

Latham, G. P., & Locke, E. a. (2009). Science and ethics: What should count as evidence against the use of goal setting? *Academy of Management Perspectives, 23*(3), 88–91. https://doi.org/10.5465/AMP.2009.43479266.

Locke, E. A., & Latham, G. P. (2006). New directions in goal-setting theory. *Current Directions in Psychological Science, 15*(5), 265–268. https://doi.org/10.1111/j.1467-8721.2006.00449.x.

Macleod, L. (2013). Making SMART goals smarter. *Physician Executive, 38*, 68–70.

Madigan, C. D., Daley, A. J., Lewis, A. L., Aveyard, P., & Jolly, K. (2015). Is self-weighing an effective tool for weight loss: a systematic literature review and meta-analysis. *International Journal of Behavioral Nutrition and Physical Activity, 12*(1), 104. https://doi.org/10.1186/s12966-015-0267-4.

Martorella, G., Côté, J., Racine, M., & Choinière, M. (2012). Web-based nursing intervention for self-management of pain after cardiac surgery: Pilot randomized controlled trial. *Journal of Medical Internet Research, 14*(6), e177. https://doi.org/10.2196/jmir.2070.

McCallum, S. (2012). Gamification and serious games for personalized health. *Studies in Health Technology and Informatics, 177*, 85–96. Retrieved from http://www.ncbi.nlm.nih.gov/pubmed/22942036.

MedicineNet. (2016). *Definition of chronic disease*. Retrieved from http://www.medicinenet.com/script/main/art.asp?articlekey=33490

Michie, S., Ashford, S., Sniehotta, F. F., Dombrowski, S. U., Bishop, A., & French, D. P. (2011). A refined taxonomy of behaviour change techniques to help people change their physical activity and healthy eating behaviours: The CALO-RE taxonomy. *Psychology and Health, 26*(11), 1479–1498. https://doi.org/10.1080/08870446.2010.540664.

Michie, S., Richardson, M., Johnston, M., Abraham, C., Francis, J., Hardeman, W., … Wood, C. E. (2013). The behavior change technique taxonomy (v1) of 93 hierarchically clustered techniques: Building an international consensus for the reporting of behavior change interventions. *Annals of Behavioral Medicine, 46*(1), 81–95. https://doi.org/10.1007/s12160-013-9486-6.

Moskowitz, G. B., & Halvorson, H. G. (2009). *The psychology of goals*. Guilford Press. Retrieved from https://www.guilford.com/books/The-Psychology-of-Goals/Moskowitz-Grant/9781606230299/reviews

Nelson, R. O. (1977). Assessment and therapeutic functions of self-monitoring. In *Progress in behaviour modification* (Vol. 5, pp. 3–41). Elsevier. https://doi.org/10.1016/B978-0-12-535605-3.50012-1.

Ness, R. B., Koopman, J. S., & Roberts, M. S. (2007). Causal system modeling in chronic disease epidemiology: A proposal. *Annals of Epidemiology, 17*(7), 564–568. https://doi.org/10.1016/j.annepidem.2006.10.014.

Nindrea, R. D., Aryandono, T., Lazuardi, L., & Dwiprahasto, I. (2018). Diagnostic accuracy of different machine learning algorithms for breast Cancer risk calculation: a meta-analysis. *Asian Pacific Journal of Cancer Prevention, 19*(7), 1747–1752. https://doi.org/10.22034/APJCP.2018.19.7.1747.

Obermayer, J. L., Riley, W. T., Asif, O., & Jean-Mary, J. (2004). College smoking-cessation using cell phone text messaging. *Journal of American College Health, 53*(2), 71–78. https://doi.org/10.3200/JACH.53.2.71-78.

Orr, J. A., & King, R. J. (2015). Mobile phone SMS messages can enhance healthy behaviour: a meta-analysis of randomised controlled trials. *Health Psychology Review, 9*, 397–416. https://doi.org/10.1080/17437199.2015.1022847.

Ovbiagele, B., Jenkins, C., Patel, S., Brunner-Jackson, B., Anderson, A., Saulson, R., & Treiber, F. (2015). Mobile health medication adherence and blood pressure control in recent stroke patients. *Journal of the Neurological Sciences, 358*, 535. https://doi.org/10.1016/j.jns.2015.10.008.

Parmar, P., Krishnamurthi, R., Ikram, M. A., Hofman, A., Mirza, S. S., Varakin, Y., … Feigin, V. L. (2015). The stroke Riskometer™ App: Validation of a data collection tool and stroke risk predictor. *International Journal of Stroke, 10*(2), 231–244. https://doi.org/10.1111/ijs.12411.

Pizzoli, S., Mazzocco, K., Triberti, S., Monzani, D., Alcañiz Raya, M. L., & Pravettoni, G. (2019). User-centered virtual reality for promoting relaxation: An innovative approach. *Frontiers in Psychology, 10*, 479. https://doi.org/10.3389/fpsyg.2019.00479.

Prochaska, J., & Diclemente, C. (1983). Stages and processes of self-change of smoking – toward an integrative model of change. *Journal of Consulting and Clinical Psychology, 51*, 390. https://doi.org/10.1037//0022-006X.51.3.390.

Prochaska, J., & Velicer, W. F. (1997). The transtheoretical model of health behavior change. *American Journal of Health Promotion, 12*(1), 38–48. https://doi.org/10.4278/0890-1171-12.1.38.

Redfern, J., Usherwood, T., Harris, M. F., Rodgers, A., Hayman, N., Panaretto, K., … Peiris, D. (2014). A randomised controlled trial of a consumer-focused e-health strategy for cardiovascular risk management in primary care: The consumer navigation of electronic cardiovascular tools (CONNECT) study protocol. *BMJ Open, 4*(2), 1–9. https://doi.org/10.1136/bmjopen-2013-004523.

Renzi, C., Riva, S., Masiero, M., & Pravettoni, G. (2016). The choice dilemma in chronic hematological conditions: Why choosing is not only a medical issue? A psycho-cognitive perspective. *Critical Reviews in Oncology/Hematology, 99*, 134. https://doi.org/10.1016/j.critrevonc.2015.12.010.

Rose, G. (1995). *The strategy of preventive medicine*. New York: Oxford University Press.

Rosenstock, I. M. (1974). Historical origins of the health belief model. *Health Education Monographs, 2*(4), 328–335.

Rubel, P., Fayn, J., Nollo, G., Assanelli, D., Li, B., Restier, L., … Chevalier, P. (2005). Toward personal eHealth in cardiology. Results from the EPI-MEDICS telemedicine project. *Journal of Electrocardiology, 38*(4), 100–106. https://doi.org/10.1016/j.jelectrocard.2005.06.011.

Rubel, P., Fayn, J., Simon-Chautemps, L., Atoui, H., Ohlsson, M., Telisson, D., … Chevalier, P. (2004). New paradigms in telemedicine: Ambient intelligence, wearable, pervasive and personalized. In *Wearable eHealth systems for personalised health management: State of the art and future challenges* (Vol. 108). Fairfax: IOS Press.

Runge, C., Lecheler, J., Horn, M., Tews, J.-T., & Schaefer, M. (2006). Outcomes of a web-based patient education program for asthmatic children and adolescents. *Chest, 129*(3), 581–593. https://doi.org/10.1378/chest.129.3.581.

Sardi, L., Idri, A., & Fernández-Alemán, J. L. (2017). A systematic review of gamification in e-health. *Journal of Biomedical Informatics, 71*, 31. https://doi.org/10.1016/j.jbi.2017.05.011.

Schwarzer, R. (1992). Self-efficacy in the adoption and maintenance of health behaviors: Theoretical approaches and a new model. In *Self-efficacy: Thought control of action*. Washington: Hemisphere.

Schwarzer, R. (2008). Modeling health behavior change: How to predict and modify the adoption and maintenance of health behaviors. *Applied Psychology, 57*(1), 1–29. https://doi.org/10.1111/j.1464-0597.2007.00325.x.

Schwarzer, R., Lippke, S., & Luszczynska, A. (2011). Mechanisms of health behavior change in persons with chronic illness or disability: The health action process approach (HAPA). *Rehabilitation Psychology, 56*(3), 161–170. https://doi.org/10.1037/a0024509.

Schweier, R., Romppel, M., Richter, C., Hoberg, E., Hahmann, H., Scherwinski, I., … Grande, G. (2014). A web-based peer-modeling intervention aimed at lifestyle changes in patients with coronary heart disease and chronic back pain: Sequential controlled trial. *Journal of Medical Internet Research, 16*(7), 1–14. https://doi.org/10.2196/jmir.3434.

Seuring, T., Archangelidi, O., & Suhrcke, M. (2015). The economic costs of type 2 diabetes: A global systematic review. *Pharmaco Economics, 33*(8), 811–831. https://doi.org/10.1007/s40273-015-0268-9.

Sharkey, A. R., & Modarai, B. (2018). Medical management of risk factors for vascular disease. *Surgery (United Kingdom), 36*(6), 265–271. https://doi.org/10.1016/j.mpsur.2018.03.007.

Singanayagam, A., Schembri, S., & Chalmers, J. D. (2013). Predictors of mortality in hospitalized adults with acute exacerbation of chronic obstructive pulmonary disease: A systematic review and meta-analysis. *Annals of the American Thoracic Society, 10*(2), 81–89. https://doi.org/10.1513/AnnalsATS.201208-043OC.

Srikesavan, C., Williamson, E., Cranston, T., Hunter, J., Adams, J., Lamb, E., & S. (2018). An online hand exercise intervention for adults with rheumatoid arthritis (mySARAH): Design, development, and usability testing. *JMIR Rehabilitation and Assistive Technologies, 20*, e10457. https://doi.org/10.2196/10457.

Steca, P., Greco, A., D'Addario, M., Monzani, D., Pozzi, R., Villani, A., … & Parati, G. (2013). Relationship of illness severity with health and life satisfaction in patients with cardiovascular disease: The mediating role of self-efficacy beliefs and illness perceptions. *Journal of Happiness Studies, 14*(5), 1585–1599.

Steca, P., Greco, A., Cappelletti, E., D'addario, M., Monzani, D., Pancani, L., … & Parati, G. (2015). Cardiovascular management self-efficacy: Psy-chometric properties of a new scale and its usefulness in a rehabilitation context. *Annals of Behavioral Medicine, 49*(5), 660–674.

Stoll, R. D., Pina, A. A., Gary, K., & Amresh, A. (2017). Usability of a smartphone application to support the prevention and early intervention of anxiety in youth. *Cognitive and Behavioral Practice, 24*, 393. https://doi.org/10.1016/j.cbpra.2016.11.002.

Strandbygaard, U., Thomsen, S. F., & Backer, V. (2010). A daily SMS reminder increases adherence to asthma treatment: A three-month follow-up study. *Respiratory Medicine, 104*(2), 166–171. https://doi.org/10.1016/j.rmed.2009.10.003.

Stroebe, W. (2011). *Social psychology and health*. McGraw-Hill Education. Retrieved from https://xpv.uab.cat/pub/quapsi/DanaInfo=.adefCyfhGkj3+02113481v12n1p7.pdf

Thissen, M., Udrea, A., Hacking, M., von Braunmuehl, T., & Ruzicka, T. (2017). mHealth app for risk assessment of pigmented and nonpigmented skin lesions—A study on sensitivity and specificity in detecting malignancy. *Telemedicine and E-Health*. https://doi.org/10.1089/tmj.2016.0259.

Tregarthen, J. P., Lock, J., & Darcy, A. M. (2015). Development of a smartphone application for eating disorder self-monitoring. *International Journal of Eating Disorders, 48*(7), 972–982. https://doi.org/10.1002/eat.22386.

Uchino, B. N., Bowen, K., Kent de Grey, R., Mikel, J., & Fisher, E. B. (2018). Social support and physical health: Models, mechanisms, and opportunities. In *Principles and concepts of behavioral medicine* (pp. 341–372). New York: Springer New York. https://doi.org/10.1007/978-0-387-93826-4_12.

Udrea, A., & Lupu, C. (2014). Real-time acquisition of quality verified nonstandardized color images for skin lesions risk assessment – A preliminary study. *2014 18th international conference on system theory, control and computing, ICSTCC 2014*, (February 2016), (pp. 199–204). https://doi.org/10.1109/ICSTCC.2014.6982415.

Van Vugt, M., De Wit, M., Cleijne, W. H. J. J., & Snoek, F. J. (2013). Use of behavioral change techniques in web-based self-management programs for type 2 diabetes patients: Systematic review. *Journal of Medical Internet Research, 15*(12), e279. https://doi.org/10.2196/jmir.2800.

Vergani, L., Marton, G., Pizzoli, S., Monzani, D., Mazzocco, K., & Pravettoni, G. (2019). Training cognitive functions using mobile apps in breast Cancer patients: Systematic review. *JMIR mHealth and uHealth, 7*(3), e10855. https://doi.org/10.2196/10855.

Villalba Mora, E., Ottaviano, M., Arredondo, M., Martinez, A., & Guillen, S. (2006). Wearable monitoring system for heart failure assessment in a mobile environment. *Computers in Cardiology, 33*, 237–240.

Villalba Mora, E., Salvi, D., Ottaviano, M., Peinado, I., Arredondo, M., & Akay, A. (2009). Wearable and mobile system to manage remotely heart failure. In *Information technology in biomedicine, IEEE transactions on* (Vol. 13). New York: Institute of Electrical and Electronics Engineers. https://doi.org/10.1109/TITB.2009.2026572.

Wantland, D. J., Portillo, C. J., Holzemer, W. L., Slaughter, R., & McGhee, E. M. (2004). The effectiveness of web-based vs. non-web-based interventions: A meta-analysis of behavioral change outcomes. *Journal of Medical Internet Research, 6*(4), e40. https://doi.org/10.2196/jmir.6.4.e40.

Webb, T. L., Joseph, J., Yardley, L., & Michie, S. (2010). Using the internet to promote health behavior change: A systematic review and meta-analysis of the impact of theoretical basis, use of behavior change techniques, and mode of delivery on efficacy. *Journal of Medical Internet Research, 12*(1), 1–18. https://doi.org/10.2196/jmir.1376.

World Health Organization. (2008a). Chronic respiratory diseases. *Aids Research Programme, 1*, 001–156. https://doi.org/10.1136/jech.47.1.4.

World Health Organization. (2008b). *The global burden of disease: Update*. Geneva: World Health Organization.

World Health Organization. (2009). *Mortality and burden of disease attributable to selected major risks*. doi:https://doi.org/10.2471/BLT.09.070565.

World Health Organization. (2015). *Integrated chronic disease prevention and control*. Retrieved October 16, 2018, from http://www.who.int/chp/about/integrated_cd/en/

World Health Organization. (2017). Progress monitor 2017. World Health Organization. Retrieved October 16, 2018, from https://apps.who.int/iris/bitstream/handle/10665/258940/9789241513029-eng.pdf;jsessionid=68B0EAA3447DE6AE4E2C20269815D6BB?sequence=1

Wu, I. X. Y., Kee, J. C. Y., Threapleton, D. E., Ma, R. C. W., Lam, V. C. K., Lee, E. K. P., … Chung, V. C. H. (2018). Effectiveness of smartphone technologies on glycaemic control in patients with type 2 diabetes: Systematic review with meta-analysis of 17 trials. *Obesity Reviews : An Official Journal of the International Association for the Study of Obesity, 19*(6), 825–838. https://doi.org/10.1111/obr.12669.

Wu, Y. P., Aspinwall, L. G., Conn, B. M., Stump, T., Grahmann, B., & Leachman, S. A. (2016). A systematic review of interventions to improve adherence to melanoma preventive behaviors for individuals at elevated risk. *Preventive Medicine, 88*, 153. https://doi.org/10.1016/j.ypmed.2016.04.010.

Yee, N., & Bailenson, J. (2007). The Proteus effect: The effect of transformed self-representation on behavior. *Human Communication Research, 33*(3), 271–290. https://doi.org/10.1111/j.1468-2958.2007.00299.x.

Zheng, Y., Klem, M. L., Sereika, S. M., Danford, C. A., Ewing, L. J., & Burke, L. E. (2015). Self-weighing in weight management: A systematic literature review. *Obesity, 23*(2), 256–265. https://doi.org/10.1002/oby.20946.

Chapter 4
An Introduction to Personalized eHealth

Valeria Sebri and Lucrezia Savioni

1 Introduction

In recent years, the field of personalized medicine has greatly expanded and has attracted great interest not only among professionals but also from the general public. The concept of "therapy for a disease" is no longer satisfactory, and the need for a drug that takes into account the individual becomes more and more a necessity (Ginsburg and Willard 2009; Plebani 2016).

However, the paradigm of personalized medicine is not new in the field of care; medicine has always taken into consideration the variability of individuals by treating the patient in relation to his/her differences both in terms of diagnosis and response to treatment; for example, blood typing has long been used to conduct blood transfusions and organ transplants (Collins and Varmus 2015).

Advancements in science and technology have allowed a more in-depth study of human genetic individuality. In particular, the enormous development of genetics, through DNA sequencing, has enabled scientists to manage a large amount of data.

Some examples are the powerful methods to characterize patients (such as different cell dosages, geomorphology, proteomics, metabolomics, and even mobile health technology), the development of large-scale biological databases (such as the human genome sequence), and computational tools for the analysis of large data sets.

All these advances, inseparable from the sociological aspects, have allowed the development of a more objective approach to diagnosis and targeted therapies and

V. Sebri (✉) · L. Savioni
Department of Oncology and Hemato-Oncology, University of Milan, Milan, Italy

Applied Research Division for Cognitive and Psychological Science,
European Institute of Oncology (IEO) IRCCS, Milan, Italy
e-mail: valeria.sebri@ieo.it; lucrezia.savioni@ieo.it

G. Pravettoni, S. Triberti (eds.), *P5 eHealth: An Agenda for the Health Technologies of the Future*, https://doi.org/10.1007/978-3-030-27994-3_4

the ability to predict the response to therapy, avoiding undesirable effects (Collins and Varmus 2015; Offit 2011). The field of oncology has derived the largest benefits from the use of personalized medicine. The application of molecular biology technology has allowed a precise distinction between the different types of cancer, an early diagnosis for some forms of cancer, and a definition of ad hoc therapeutic strategies for the cancer patient.

1.1 What Are the News of Personalized Medicine?

Compared to "traditional" medicine, personalized medicine allows greater precision in predicting risk and responding to therapies (Ginsburg and Willard 2009; Swan 2009; Zhang et al. 2012).

The result is P5 approach, a model of healthcare based on proactive (preventive) planning (cfr. Chap. 3), unlike the traditional model of reactive health (episodic). Indeed, traditional medicine interventions were implemented in acute crisis, i.e., when the disease was already established and sometimes irreversible. Furthermore, disease treatment and prevention strategies are developed for the general population, without distinction. We then move from a one-dimensional clinical approach to one focused on the patient, in order to optimize medical decisions and to apply specific treatments.

1.2 A Brief History

As previously mentioned, personalized medicine is a known field. Since ancient times, doctors were convinced that the onset of diseases had different causes. They believed that subjects with the same disease should be treated differently from one another because of the physical and psychic differences.

Previously, the Egyptians distinguished the endogenous causes (corruption of the intestinal contents due to a "matter pecans"), the exogenous causes (natural calamities, parasites, bites of animals), the hidden causes (revenge of a dead person, wrath of God, hatred of enemies), and finally the psychogenic causes (mood disorders or psychosomatic pathologies).

Subsequently, Hippocrates (480–390 b.c.) began to take care of the ill person and not of the disease (Grmek 1993), considering alimentation, physical activity, lifestyle, and climate. Hippocrates unifies "in a critical analysis the patient, the sickness, the physician and above all proposes the integration of the physical and psychological uniqueness of the subject with the socio-cultural and physical-geographical complexity of his environment" (Zitelli and Palmer 1979). Claudio Galeno introduced the concept of predisposition (129–200 a.c.). Taking up the humoral theory of Hippocrates, he introduced two internal causes beside the body's external causes:

- Causes that predispose a certain individual to certain diseases
- Immediate causes that the doctor can only see when the disease has started

Galeno also expanded this theory to the healing of the patient; he argues that healing from an illness also depends heavily on the patient's life habits (alimentation, rest, sexual activity, emotional state). According to this theory "the patient needs individualized attention, since the preservation of health changes according to the complexions and bodily habitus" (Sotres 1993).

More recently, Sacks dealt with this theme. He showed that patients with the same disease are fundamentally different from each other and that the technical-scientific evaluations were insufficient because they "revealed only the deficits and not the abilities; they provide us only fragmentary data and patterns, while we need to see a music, a story, a series of actions lived" (Sacks 1986). For example, he mentions that patients with Tourette syndrome were never the same.

The development of technologies and the progress of science have today led to the study of interindividual variability through genotypic characteristics. The discovery and study of the human genome has allowed an incredible advancement of personalized medicine. Although personalized medicine is an area that has always been known and it is an intuitive concept, there are different opinions about its definition. In fact, today there is not yet a precise and universally accepted definition of personalized medicine (Table 4.1).

In Table 4.2 instead, we compare the five main definitions of personalized medicine. The first one by Carlson (2008) considers the prevention and treatment of disease based on the patient's genetic profile. Differently, Personalized Medicine Coalition's definition considers prevention as predisposition of patients to particular disease and the management of illness.

The definition from the America Medical Association is only about pharmacological treatment. Finally, the third definition gives information about prevention, treatment, and individuality.

As we can see, psychological aspects are considered by only one definition (Personalized Medicine Coalition's definition). As we saw before, personalized medicine uses the information about patient's life, to create an individualized care and cure (cfr. Chap. 1). It is fundamental to consider that the patient's life is

Table 4.1 Personalized medicine definitions

Definition	Reference
Prevention, diagnosis, and therapy of a specific disease based on the individual genetic profile	Carlson (2008)
Use of new methods of molecular analysis to better manage an illness or the predisposition to pathologies	Personalized Medicine Coalition
Provide the right treatment to the right patient at the right dose	European Union
Medicine based on the clinical, genetic, and environmental information of each person	American Medical Association
Medicine that uses information about genes, proteins, and the person's environment to prevent, diagnose, and treat diseases	National Cancer Institute

Table 4.2 The definition of personalized medicine on comparison

Definition	Prevention	Treatment	Individuality	Psychological aspects
Carlson (2008)	x	x	x	–
Personalized Medicine Coalition	x	–	–	x
European Union	–	x	–	–
American Medical Association	–	–	x	–
National Cancer Institute	x	x	x	–

constituted not only by genomic aspects but also by his social condition, work (activity), family history, etc. (cfr. Chap. 3).

This underlines the confusion surrounding the definition of personalized medicine.

In general, personalized medicine can be defined as the medical approach that uses the specific biological characteristics, environment, needs, and lifestyle of an individual to create ad hoc therapy, including drugs, dosages, and other possible remedies (Swan 2009; Capurso 2018; Jameson and Longo 2015).

2 The Development of Personalized Medicine

The development of personalized medicine and the increased knowledge between genes and external factors have brought some changes in different fields of healthcare:

- Treatments
- Diagnosis and risk prediction
- Doctor-patient communication
- Disease/illness management

Further, we will analyze them one by one to better understand how and what are the changes that personalized medicine has brought in each of these areas.

2.1 Treatments

From the earliest times, it was known that the response to drugs is genetically determined. Over the years, we have seen how, together with its genetic heritage, other factors play a fundamental role, including health status, environmental exposure, nutrition, and age (cfr. Chap. 3).

The introduction of personalized medicine has allowed the extension of the approaches traditionally used for the understanding and treatment of diseases (Vogenberg et al. 2010; Ginsburg and Willard 2009).

Thus, pharmacogenomics was born, a discipline that consists in the study of genomic characteristics that determine individual differences in the response to drugs; it has allowed doctors to select drugs and to create customized intervention protocols on the nature of diseases, diagnosis, responses to treatments, and its individual characteristics (Panahiazar et al. 2014). Pharmacogenomics allows the following:

- The prediction of possible side effects of drugs on specific patients
- The identification of the susceptibility of an individual to certain diseases, allowing doctors to draw up a monitoring and prevention plan
- To define a priori the best treatment and the best drugs for specific patients

Doctors will be able to make more effective clinical decisions for each patient, going beyond the classic "one-size-fits-all" concept.

The personalization of treatments also allows identifying the subpopulations that behave differently toward a given drug, compared to the typical patient. This creates more stringent inclusion/exclusion criteria that make treatment positive in terms of safety and efficacy (Richmond 2008).

2.2 *Diagnosis and Risk Prediction*

The progress of genomics has allowed, through the execution of genetic tests, the identification of genomic alterations that underlies many genetic diseases. This allows to obtain information on the probability that an individual can develop a disease, especially the most difficult to treat, such as cancer, diabetes, or cardiovascular disorders. In this way, doctors will be able to develop individual interventions to avoid or control the development of the pathology, by implementing, for example, changes in the patient's lifestyle (cfr. Chap. 3) (Steffen and Lenz 2013; Gaitskell 2017).

In this way, we can focus more on prevention rather than on the management of the disease (cfr. Chap. 3). With this aim, we can, in the future, use the collection of genetic information from prenatal tests, to outline possible diseases that can be avoided or adequately controlled.

The use of personalized medicine in the field of prevention, and also in P5 approach, can therefore significantly reduce the incidence of diseases, especially chronic ones. However, the development of biological markers based on primary prevention is still distant, despite the enormous development of research (Panahiazar et al. 2014; Katsios and Roukos 2010).

2.3 Doctor-Patient Communication

With the introduction of personalized medicine, there will be more and more information about the available treatment options, to be understood and discussed by the patient and the doctor. This implies a change in the relationship and, in particular, in the patient-doctor communication. The doctor-patient communication concerns two subjects who are in an unfair and often in a not voluntary position. Both patient and the physician find themselves in difficulty: the patient, following a diagnosis, finds himself in a state of shock and refusal that makes it difficult to process the information that is provided or does not have the necessary knowledge to understand them; on the other hand, the doctor often lacks the confidence and training necessary to provide patients with clear, understandable, and empathetic information and finds himself having to conduct the interview quickly and in an unsuitable place. In this situation very often the patient's expectations or understandings are left in the background, focusing only on the biomedical aspects (Kerr et al. 2003; Ong et al. 1995). The introduction of personalized medicine implies a change in the relationship and, in particular, in the patient-doctor communication. Communication must be characterized by three key elements shared by both parties:

- Information
- Autonomy
- Responsibility

In accordance with P5 approach, this means that the professional will aim to create a more personalized environment that promotes the flow of information; communication will be more informative: the specialist will tend to be more clear, using a colloquial language that is understandable for the patient and will provide such information with empathy, dignity, and respect. In this way, the whole process of diagnosis and treatment is clear and understandable. At the same time, the patient will feel more involved and no longer a passive subject (cfr. Chap. 1); he will be able to express his preferences on treatments, for example, he will be able to have a say in the choice of treatment planning or in the choice of the various exercises proposed, etc.. In this way, the doctor will no longer feel the only responsible for the outcome of the intervention, but a sharing of responsibility is established (Lemay et al. 2017; Cutica et al. 2014).

2.4 Disease/Illness Management

The change in communication between doctor and patient has made healthcare more collaborative, allowing patients to be participants and guides of their path to recovery (Gorini et al. 2018). The involvement of the patient in the decision-making process recognizes the autonomy of the latter, who will be more inclined to accept and follow the treatment leading to the possibility of a better prognosis (Cutica et al.

2014). The patient's knowledge of his condition will lead to more and more experienced and more active patients managing their pathology in the future, which is the purpose of P5 approach.

In the future, the patient-driven medicine could expedite dramatically the clinical trial process. Health social networks can bring standardized digital data and pre-aggregated patient registries to clinical trial conductors. Moreover, a collaboration between health social networks and clinical trial representatives can be created, on their needs for electronic data collection, ensuring that the quantitative information necessary for clinical trials is already available to all participating patients. Clinical trial prescreening survey can be administered easily through health social network websites (Swan 2009).

3 The Role of eHealth (and mHealth Specifically)

Considering the complexity of eHealth resources (cfr. Chap. 1), we will focus on mHealth, which is characterized by technologies particularly useful for the aim of personalization.

When we speak about mHealth, we refer to mobile telecommunication technologies supporting wellness through the delivery of healthcare (Steinhubl et al. 2013; Gorini et al. 2018; Triberti et al. 2019).

The smartphone could become the hub of future medicine, also regarding mental health services (Ben-Zeev et al. 2013). Personalized medicine in P5 approach includes for example the possibility to access *real-time patient self-report data* (cfr. Chap. 3) during the time interval between visits. In other words, eHealth could be a support for patients and caregivers in terms of self-monitoring. Mobile phones and other personal devices indeed can improve the accessibility to these data sets. Indeed, these can be utilized in order to help patients in gathering information about their own diseases so to make them able to manage their own situation more effectively.

Iterative development processes could create applications that will be available on multiple platforms (cfr. Chap 9), used also to improve patients' acceptance of disease in often complicated day-to-day routines (Diamantidis and Becker 2014). Patients could have access to data collection, becoming active managers of their symptoms, potentially leading to more accurate assessment. Berrouiguet et al. (2018) describe an example in which eHealth tools allow an endocrinologist to chart blood glucose levels. In this way, before and after a doctor's appointment, health professionals could observe and control these values with a portable blood glucose meter. At the same time, changes in sleep, appetite, mood, and other behavioral and psychological data could be recorded, which is important both for physical and mental health management. In general, smartphones and portable computers have a pluripotent impact in terms of collection of data about blood pressure, glucose, brain waves, and heart rhythm.

Therefore, we can observe an interesting aspect in P5 approach: patients could update their data in order to *be carried on by medical staff* in each moment of the day; at the same time, the combination of real-time self-monitoring and contextual information could enhance medical decision-making, according to data analysis tools. Data can be collected by patients or caregivers themselves, and they could be reported in a portable device or could be captured through sensors in the patient's living environment. The choice and challenge of using artificial intelligence data-mining techniques give the possibility for improving clinical decision-making and a more personalized treatment (Van der Krieke et al. 2013; Durand et al. 2014; Gorini et al. 2018). In addition, it is possible to *reduce the number of visits to the doctor*. Many measurements will be acquired by oneself; people will collect data also respecting their own convenience, and it is possible to assume that much more information will be acquired than ever before (Van Dyck et al. 2016; Steinberg et al. 2013).

eHealth could become an *instrument of cost reduction and prevention* (cfr. Chap. 1); the idea is that this technology will be developed with the aim of leading a reduction in resource consumption, emergency room use, and number of patients recovering in hospitals. Indeed, the delocalization of therapeutic procedures permitted by the use of mobile-based resources will make possible to reduce the necessity for the patients to reach the hospital for any healthcare need. This would be desirable also in terms of keeping away infections and other problems related to recovery in hospitals (Hayes et al. 2014). For example, the high risk of social isolation caused by recovery could increase delays in patients' discharges from care hospitals (Landeiro et al. 2016). Possibly, hospital recovery will be necessary only in specific conditions; it will be part of an important change; for all other cases, patients will be taken care of at their homes, with the help of mobile healthcare technologies. These instruments can also answer to the emergence of new treatment paradigms able to determine when a disease is a current or a future burden for someone, with the desire to anticipate illness and its consequences (preventive medicine) (Rotily and Roze 2013) (see Fig. 4.1).

It is clear that the importance of safety and regulation of smartphone apps in this advancing field is in continuous growth, aiming to an accurate and meticulous sharing of a person's care (Hayes et al. 2014), which also raises ethical issues such as privacy concerns (cfr. Chap. 10). A future perspective of eHealth-related personalized medicine could include the role of caregivers. Family members and friends are an important form of support for patients (cfr. Chap. 3); in this sense, eHealth could become a key facilitator of medical adherence helping unprepared people for the demand of caring. Technologies indeed could require support and training in the process of caring (Car et al. 2017). In addition, in the future we could assume the ongoing growth of new services based on a user-centered approach and iterative development processes, even evaluating the context of use (Scandurra and Sjölinder 2013) (cfr. Chap. 9).

Another interesting resource for personalization among digital technologies (relating both mobile and non-mobile devices) regards *avatars*. Avatars are digital representations of users within digital environments, ranging from static images (e.g., in social networks) to dynamic figures able to act and move (e.g., in video games). Avatars are often customized by users, and according to literature, such customization

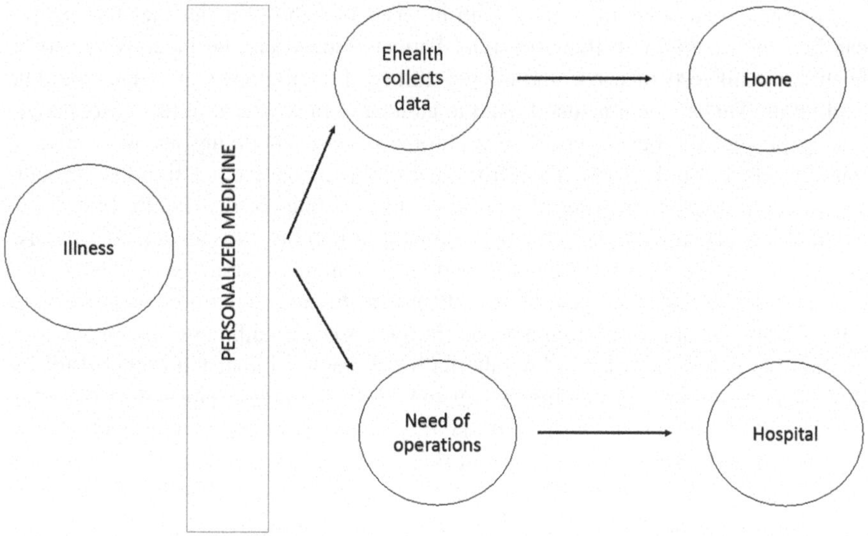

Fig. 4.1 The impact of personalized medicine on hospitalization

process is not random, rather users tend to use avatars to represent aspects of their physical appearance, personality, and even beliefs in a symbolic manner.

In that some eHealth technologies entail social network features or video games/serious games, avatars can appear in this field. An interesting development is to exploit this specific feature beyond its basic representational features; creating dynamical avatars whose appearance changes over time depending on users' behavior (e.g., adherence to therapy and to healthy activities) would create a digital feedback of patients' progress through their own healthcare journey (Triberti and Chirico 2017).

Moreover, recent studies are exploring the idea that digital avatars created by patients could be analyzed such as drawings and personal artifacts, in that they may be characterized by relevant features to be considered for psychological assessment (e.g., patients with low self-esteem and depression symptoms may create less detailed avatars) (Triberti et al. 2017; Villani et al. 2016).

Indeed, giving patients the opportunity to represent themselves is another resource both in terms of engagement and self-expression and also an innovative source of health-related information for health providers and researchers.

4 Liability: The Road Toward Becoming Active Patients

During the specification of technologies referring to P5 approach, we cannot forget an important included aspect: *the sense of liability*. Technologies in general, and also eHealth, should include a reflection on this ethic element because the usage of these instruments has both benefits and limits.

Firstly, a great advantage of eHealth in terms of liability underlines that people can become *healthier* in their lifestyle. Patients indeed can be incentivized to be healthier in all sorts of ways, and the possibility of having one's own data could be a stimulus. This concept is also linked to an idea of prevention; in this case, people ideally prevent the development of a chronic disease, involving an own sense of liability (Hayes et al. 2014). Therefrom, liability is a positive reaction that an individual could improve in front of a possible disease, helped by eHealth. In order to explain how eHealth can help the development of liability, we can consider the use of genomic markers for personalized medicine. Genomic markers should be a great way in order to underline people at high risk of the more common side effects or with a high probability of nonresponse. In this case, eHealth could be an accurate and current helper in order to find alternative strategies: either with other drugs or through preventive means, including diet and physical exercise (Norman et al. 2007).

The overall goal is based on the possibility to have patients even more characterized by an *increase in level of information flow, transparency, and collaboration with personal care as well as quantitative, predictive, and preventive aspects that are basic conditions for taking responsibility* as P5 approach underlines. This idea is sustained by the current and continuous expansion of the healthcare through new services. About this, Swan (2009) underlines that social networks are a potential instrument in the field of health. Through social networks, everyone can share information and knowledge about conditions, symptoms, and treatments, creating a platform for discussion about different issues; if I would have the possibility to know my symptoms, I can prevent chronic disease or monitor a future state of illness (cfr. Chap. 3). In addition, I can read and understand similar experiences of others; patients have to accept a radical change: the repositioning from being a minimally informed advice recipient to become an active manager of their own health.

Everyone has the liability of their health, and evaluating this fundamental role, individuals must become instigating collaborators, peer leaders, and information sharers in participative medicine. In other words, liability through eHealth can bring to a transition from paternalistic healthcare to partnership models (Townsend et al. 2015). In this way, individuals become more and more engaged in the course of their care, for example, by participating in a variety of self-testing and self-management activities and becoming more and more aware of the personal and environmental factors that impact their health (Swan 2009).

Liability should not only increase in patients but also in physicians, which are active protagonists of a care co-building. If patients will be more careful about the management of their symptoms, *physicians should adapt their behavior and workout strategies* to this new shift, starting to become a care consultant and collaborator for patients. This possibility prefigures a collaboration between patients and medical staff (Appelboom et al. 2014).

In summary, eHealth could be a basic condition to supply people with personalized data for better quantification of their wellness by involving a sense of liability; individuals are more likely to have positive behavioral changes, becoming active protagonists of their life and not passive recipients of others' decisions (Flores et al. 2013).

5 Communication Through eHealth

Genetic and genomic technologies were the start for the development of many medical specialties involved in personalized medicine. This is indeed the strategy to reduce disjointed or uncoordinated clinical care, in order to *optimize effective communication*. The overall goal aims at the promotion of patients' understanding and engagement regarding the need, and the consequent use, for these services. An interpersonal approach can also optimize the quality of care starting from the minimization of duplicate testing, providing accurate information to patients and their families and reducing gaps in healthcares. This can be the optimal result to achieve when different medical care roles will collaborate and communicate correctly with each other. This way, healthcare services can work together with patients to address all issues in a cohesive manner (Haga et al. 2015), moving to a co-diagnosis and a co-care model between physicians, patients, and other parties.

We could assist to a *change of mental representation* within the P5 approach; a collaborative communication could start to make physician a colleague and advisor, as one of many sources during a care plan. At the same time, patients could become more and more of an informed participant, an active responsibility taker, and a coordinator of his/her health program and health data (Hood and Friend 2011). Future interactions will be focused on this new way of communication: in this case, patients will call physicians in order to have a consultative co-interpretation of the results, bringing quantitative reports from their self-testing and self-tracking activities hold through eHealth services. Speaking about a change of communication, another option is to assume that could be the emergence of on-demand web-based physician consultation services with video and chat (Swan 2009).

The usage of eHealth has benefits and limitations at the same time. Several advantages of eHealth are evident starting from the high flexibility in its usage regarding *time and place*. Patients could formulate questions and understand responses in each moment through communication with healthcare professionals. We assume that eHealth could potentially contribute to an increased *quality of care* in front of the *new awareness of patients* themselves.

At the same time, if many studies underline the positive attitude of patients toward self-management, others report to patients' *feeling of inability* to judge the seriousness of their side effects and symptoms. A research of Schulman-Green et al. (2011) establishes the necessity of the assessment related to patients' preferences and ability to self-manage over time, putting attention during transitions and its possible changes.

Other limits in the use of eHealth could be patient's *age and different cancer diagnosis*. Regarding the first point, Schulman-Green et al. (2011) underline that higher age is associated with lower eHealth usage. It is also possible that the number of comorbidity conditions in older persons influences self-management ability negatively. Variations toward eHealth among different cancer diagnosis groups are instead examined in depth by Boyes et al. (2012); they report that prostate and testicular cancer survivors had a more positive attitude toward online contact with healthcare professionals. It's clear the preference to *communicate online intimate symptoms encountered*, such as incontinence, infertility, and reduced sexual functioning. Børøsund et al. (2013) describe different attitudes toward eHealth between breast and prostate cancer patients; *sex* is in fact another important element of discussion. Among women with breast cancer, high use of eHealth is typical of those with depression and low levels of perceived social support; for men with prostate cancer, eHealth's usage is instead linked to symptom distress. In another study (Triberti et al. 2018), males were more likely to use mobile app's notes function to communicate with the health providers, both in terms of medical information and personal confidences, comments, and emotional states.

As a solution, future eHealth and mHealth resources should be designed basing on users' personal characteristics, desires, and contexts, in order to tailor such devices and services on their own predispositions; according to literature, this would augment the probability that such solutions will be accepted and productively used (cfr. Chap 9).

6 Health Social Networks

In this chapter, we have had the occasion to discover how eHealth (mobile technologies and social networks specifically) can support the introduction of personalized medicine in the P5 approach. It is important to focus on social networks in order to provide more details on how this important resource of web-based technologies can be used within a P5 approach to healthcare:

1. Health social networks are primarily directed to patients, but, at the same time, we know that caretakers, families, and other interested parties may be involved (Gage-Bouchard et al. 2017). Sharing information and emotional support is important in order to build networks of relationships, reducing the idea to be lonely during the healthcare process.
2. Several health social networks (e.g., eHealth forum) give the possibility to pose some questions to physicians (Hawn 2009). This transparency changes the image of doctors: it is not a 10-min accessible collaborator in care, but it could become a professional role based on the willingness to interact with patients. Even this basic mechanism of lightweight doctor-patient interaction could change burdens on the healthcare system.
3. eHealth forum could also be used in order to create a community with other patients in which feeling of commonality and mutual comprehension are presented. This eHealth forum offers the sharing of feelings and personal opinions that could be useful for patients lacking social relationships or having the need to speak with other people with their same medical condition (Nabi et al. 2013).
4. Another type of service offered by health social networks is based on quantified self-tracking, that is, an easy-to-use data entry screening for symptoms, treatments, and other biological information (Aral and Nicolaides 2017; Morris and

Aguilera 2012). The use of graphical displays or other strategies could improve patient's ability of understanding treatments, in order to become active protagonists of their cares and, eventually, to be able to call physicians if there is a negative symptom of disease. This object aims at a personalized medicine based on prevention.

5. In addition, regarding the importance of scientific publications, we could assume the possibility to use information for clinical trials. The availability of large searchable online databases in which health history and condition information of patients are included could improve traditional clinical trials, making them more efficient (Groves et al. 2013).

7 Challenges to eHealth Usages and Possible Solutions

New health technologies (eHealth) are recognized as having a major impact on health promotion and management. These tools allow to develop the implementation of integrated, sustainable, and patient-centered services and to promote an effective exchange between patient and doctor, with the patient acquiring an active role in the health process (Barello et al. 2016; Gorini et al. 2018). However, in some cases, eHealth is often unacceptable and/or long term adopted by its users.

There are many factors that can influence the use of eHealth to monitor patient health. Firstly, in some patients the idea of being constantly monitored can create excessive anxiety; in fact, patients with low self-control, through the use of self-monitored technologies, may be afraid of having more problems or treatments for the well-being of patients (Kessel et al. 2017). If the patient is not convinced of the usefulness of these tools for his health management, or if he/she is excessively afraid of the disease, such new commitments could be a source of further stress and negative attitude treatment comparisons. In such situations, patients can not only abandon the eHealth tools but also their trust in healthcare professionals can be reduced with detrimental effects on the effectiveness of the health management process as a whole.

In most cases, considering eHealth not useful for oneself, it is related to the lack of customization of the tools. The functions and contents of eHealth (including required information, patient feedback, etc.) should be adapted to the patient's individual biopsychosocial characteristics to provide more useful, more accepted, and nonredundant information (Gorini et al. 2015; Pravettoni et al. 2016). Furthermore, the personalization factors also refer to the possibility of the patient to express himself within the use of the technology. For example, eHealth functions, as well as automatic communications, will not be generalized to patient populations, but will be based on individual characteristics.

Secondly, some patients were concerned about the implementation of eHealth as a result of the budget cuts being treated. The need for face-to-face contact with professional figures is always a very requested and reassuring aspect for patients

(Mattsson et al. 2017). It is important to explain the reason for using eHealth, which is intended to accompany the work of physician and not to replace it.

In conclusion, the goal of personalized medicine, and the specific approach of P5, is to highlight the importance of a personalized technology for each type of patient.

8 Conclusion

In recent years, personalized medicine has attracted great interest and has expanded more and more, involving different areas of healthcare. In particular, it allowed changes in the choice of treatment through pharmacogenomics. Through this discipline, it has indeed been possible to predict the possible side effects of drugs on individual patients, define a priori the best treatment and the best drugs that fit the specific patient, and identify the susceptibility of an individual to certain diseases, favoring the identification of a preventive treatment plan.

All these aspects have favored the shift of attention more on prevention than the treatment of diseases. The use of personalized medicine in the field of prevention can significantly reduce the incidence of diseases, especially chronic ones.

Another aspect that has been involved since the advent of personalized medicine is the communication between doctor and patient. The doctor is more attentive to the needs of the patient, providing clear information about diagnosis and treatment. At the same time, the patient has a voice in relation to the decisions that determine their state of health and their care.

The patient is no longer a passive subject, but becomes an active one, both in decision-making and in the management of his illness. This aspect is favored by technology that through different devices has made it easier to monitor your health and communication.

eHealth, for example, could be a useful instrument for helping monitoring and managing diseases. eHealth, indeed, makes it possible for patients to be carried by medical staff in each moment of day through the combination of real-time self-monitoring with many contextual information. The result of this health strategy can enhance medical decision-making, in combination to data analysis tools. This not only brings to a reduction of the number of times patients have to visit the doctor but also is a means of reducing costs and healthcare service prevention. At the same time, as well as known, putting patients at the center of their medical care is essential for their sense of participation. It could be interesting also for increasing the sense of liability of patients through a new awareness. A collaborative communication could start to make the physician a colleague and advisor, one of many sources during a care plan. In conclusion, personalized medicine as aspect of the P5 approach is a great strategy of intervention for increasing personal skills of illness management.

Acknowledgment Valeria Sebri and Lucrezia Savioni are PhD students within the European School of Molecular Medicine (SEMM).

References

Appelboom, G., Camacho, E., Abraham, M. E., Bruce, S. S., Dumont, E. L., Zacharia, B. E., … Connolly, E. S. (2014). Smart wearable body sensors for patient self-assessment and monitoring. *Archives of Public Health, 72*(1), 28.

Aral, S., & Nicolaides, C. (2017). Exercise contagion in a global social network. *Nature Communications, 8*, 14753.

Barello, S., Triberti, S., Graffigna, G., Libreri, C., Serino, S., Hibbard, J., & Riva, G. (2016). eHealth for patient engagement: A systematic review. *Frontiers in Psychology, 6*, 2013.

Ben-Zeev, D., Davis, K. E., Kaiser, S., Krzsos, I., & Drake, R. E. (2013). Mobile technologies among people with serious mental illness: Opportunities for future services. *Administration and Policy in Mental Health and Mental Health Services Research, 40*(4), 340–343.

Berrouiguet, S., Perez-Rodriguez, M. M., Larsen, M., Baca-García, E., Courtet, P., & Oquendo, M. (2018). From eHealth to iHealth: Transition to participatory and personalized medicine in mental health. *Journal of Medical Internet Research, 20*(1), e2.

Børøsund, E., Cvancarova, M., Ekstedt, M., Moore, S. M., & Ruland, C. M. (2013). How user characteristics affect use patterns in web-based illness management support for patients with breast and prostate cancer. *Journal of Medical Internet Research, 15*(3), e34.

Boyes, A. W., Girgis, A., D'Este, C., & Zucca, A. C. (2012). Prevalence and correlates of cancer survivors' supportive care needs 6 months after diagnosis: A population-based cross-sectional study. *BMC Cancer, 12*(1), 150.

Capurso, L. (2018). Evidence-based medicine vs medicina personalizzata. *Recenti Progressi in Medicina, 109*(1), 10–14.

Car, J., Tan, W. S., Huang, Z., Sloot, P., & Franklin, B. D. (2017). eHealth in the future of medications management: Personalization, monitoring and adherence. *BMC Medicine, 15*(1), 73.

Carlson, B. (2008). What the devil is personalized medicine? *Biotechnology Healthcare, 5*(1), 17.

Collins, F. S., & Varmus, H. (2015). A new initiative on precision medicine. *New England Journal of Medicine, 372*(9), 793–795.

Cutica, I., Mc Vie, G., & Pravettoni, G. (2014). Personalized medicine: The cognitive side of patients. *European Journal of Internal Medicine, 25*(8), 685–688.

Diamantidis, C. J., & Becker, S. (2014). Health information technology (IT) to improve the care of patients with chronic kidney disease (CKD). *BMC Nephrology, 15*(1), 7.

Durand, M. A., Carpenter, L., Dolan, H., Bravo, P., Mann, M., Bunn, F., & Elwyn, G. (2014). Do interventions designed to support shared decision-making reduce health inequalities? A systematic review and meta-analysis. *PLoS One, 9*(4), e94670.

European Commision. https://ec.europa.eu/research/health/index.cfm?pg=policy&policyname=personalised

Flores, M., Glusman, G., Brogaard, K., Price, N. D., & Hood, L. (2013). P4 medicine: How systems medicine will transform the healthcare sector and society. *Personalized Medicine, 10*(6), 565–576.

Gage-Bouchard, E. A., LaValley, S., Mollica, M., & Beaupin, L. K. (2017). Cancer communication on social media: Examining how cancer caregivers use Facebook for cancer-related communication. *Cancer Nursing, 40*(4), 332–338.

Gaitskell, K. (2017). Personalised medicine approaches to screening and prevention. *The New Bioethics, 23*(1), 21–29.

Ginsburg, G. S., & Willard, H. F. (2009). Genomic and personalized medicine: Foundations and applications. *Translational Research, 154*(6), 277–287.

Gorini, A., Mazzocco, K., Gandini, S., Munzone, E., McVie, G., & Pravettoni, G. (2015). Development and psychometric testing of a breast cancer patient-profiling questionnaire. *Breast Cancer: Targets and Therapy, 7*, 133.

Gorini, A., Mazzocco, K., Triberti, S., Sebri, V., Savioni, L., & Pravettoni, G. (2018). A P5 approach to m-health: Development guidelines for advanced mobile health technology. *Frontiers in Psychology, 9*, 2066.

Grmek, M. (1993). *Storia del pensiero medico occidentale. 1. Antichità e medioevo*. Bari: Laterza.

Groves, P., Kayyali, B., Knott, D., & Van Kuiken, S. (2013). The 'big data' revolution in healthcare. *The McKinsey Quarterly, 2*(3).

Haga, S. B., Mills, R., Aucoin, J., & Taekman, J. (2015). Interprofessional education for personalized medicine through technology-based learning. *Personalized Medicine, 12*(3), 237–243.

Hawn, C. (2009). Take two aspirin and tweet me in the morning: How Twitter, Facebook, and other social media are reshaping health care. *Health Affairs, 28*(2), 361–368.

Hayes, D. F., Markus, H. S., Leslie, R. D., & Topol, E. J. (2014). Personalized medicine: Risk prediction, targeted therapies and mobile health technology. *BMC Medicine, 12*(1), 37.

Hood, L., & Friend, S. H. (2011). Predictive, personalized, preventive, participatory (P4) cancer medicine. *Nature Reviews Clinical Oncology, 8*(3), 184.

Jameson, J. L., & Longo, D. L. (2015). Precision medicine–personalized, problematic, and promising. *The New England Journal of Medicine, 372*, 2229–2234.

Katsios, C., & Roukos, D. H. (2010). Individual genomes and personalized medicine: Life diversity and complexity. *Personalized Medicine, 7*(4), 347–350.

Kerr, J., Engel, J., Schlesinger-Raab, A., Sauer, H., & Holzel, D. (2003). Doctor-patient communication. *Diseases of the Colon & Rectum, 46*(8), 1038–1046.

Kessel, K. A., Vogel, M. M., Kessel, C., Bier, H., Biedermann, T., Friess, H., … Keller, U. (2017). Mobile health in oncology: A patient survey about app-assisted cancer care. *JMIR mHealth and uHealth, 5*(6), e81.

Landeiro, F., Leal, J., & Gray, A. M. (2016). The impact of social isolation on delayed hospital discharges of older hip fracture patients and associated costs. *Osteoporosis International, 27*(2), 737–745.

Lemay, V., Hamet, P., Hizel, C., Lemarié, É., & Tremblay, Y. (2017). Personalized medicine: Interdisciplinary perspective, world tidal wave, and potential growth for the emerging countries. In *Progress and challenges in precision medicine* (pp. 301–314). Amsterdam/Boston: Elseiver/Academic.

Mattsson, S., Olsson, E. M. G., Johansson, B., & Carlsson, M. (2017). Health-related internet use in people with cancer: Results from a cross-sectional study in two outpatient clinics in Sweden. *Journal of Medical Internet Research, 19*(5), e163.

Morris, M. E., & Aguilera, A. (2012). Mobile, social, and wearable computing and the evolution of psychological practice. *Professional Psychology: Research and Practice, 43*(6), 622.

Nabi, R. L., Prestin, A., & So, J. (2013). Facebook friends with (health) benefits? Exploring social network site use and perceptions of social support, stress, and Well-being. *Cyberpsychology, Behavior and Social Networking, 16*(10), 721–727.

National Cancer Institute. http://www.cancer.gov/publications/dictionaries/cancer-terms?CdrID=561717

Norman, G. J., Zabinski, M. F., Adams, M. A., Rosenberg, D. E., Yaroch, A. L., & Atienza, A. A. (2007). A review of eHealth interventions for physical activity and dietary behavior change. American journal of preventive medicine, 33(4), 336–345

Offit, K. (2011). Personalized medicine: New genomics, old lessons. *Human Genetics, 130*(1), 3–14.

Ong, L. M., De Haes, J. C., Hoos, A. M., & Lammes, F. B. (1995). Doctor-patient communication: A review of the literature. *Social Science & Medicine, 40*(7), 903–918.

Panahiazar, M., Taslimitehrani, V., Jadhav, A., & Pathak, J. (2014, October). Empowering personalized medicine with big data and semantic web technology: Promises, challenges, and use cases. In *Big Data (Big Data), 2014 IEEE international conference on* (pp. 790–795). IEEE.

Plebani, M. (2016). Personalized medicine and clinical laboratories: Challenges and opportunities. *Biochimica Clinica, 40*(1), 33–39.

PMC Personalized Medicine Coalition. http://www.personalizedmedicinecoalition.org/science-policy/personalmed-101_overview.php.

Pravettoni, G., Mazzocco, K., Gorini, A., & Curigliano, G. (2016). Understanding cognitive processes behind acceptance or refusal of phase I trials. *Critical Reviews in Oncology/Hematology, 100*, 69–73.

Richmond, T. D. (2008). The current status and future potential of personalized diagnostics: Streamlining a customized process. *Biotechnology Annual Review, 14*, 411–422.

Rotily, M., & Roze, S. (2013). What is the impact of disease prevalence upon health technology assessment? *Best Practice & Research Clinical Gastroenterology, 27*(6), 853–865.

Sacks, O. (1986). *L'uomo che scambiò sua moglie per un cappello* (p. 240). Adelphi: Milano.

Scandurra, I., & Sjölinder, M. (2013). Participatory design with seniors: Design of future services and iterative refinements of interactive eHealth services for old citizens. *Medicine 2.0, 2*(2), e12.

Schulman-Green, D., Bradley, E. H., Knobf, M. T., Prigerson, H., Di Giovanna, M. P., & McCorkle, R. (2011). Self-management and transitions in women with advanced breast cancer. *Journal of Pain and Symptom Management, 42*(4), 517–525.

Sotres, P. G. (1993). Le regole della salute. *Storia del pensiero medico occidentale, 1*, 399–438.

Steffen, J. A., & Lenz, C. (2013). Technological evolution of diagnostic testing in oncology. *Personalized Medicine, 10*(3), 275–283.

Steinberg, D. M., Tate, D. F., Bennett, G. G., Ennett, S., Samuel-Hodge, C., & Ward, D. S. (2013). The efficacy of a daily self-weighing weight loss intervention using smart scales and e-mail. *Obesity, 21*(9), 1789–1797.

Steinhubl, S. R., Muse, E. D., & Topol, E. J. (2013). Can mobile health technologies transform health care? *JAMA, 310*(22), 2395–2396.

Swan, M. (2009). Emerging patient-driven health care models: An examination of health social networks, consumer personalized medicine and quantified self-tracking. *International Journal of Environmental Research and Public Health, 6*(2), 492–525.

Townsend, A., Leese, J., Adam, P., McDonald, M., Li, L. C., Kerr, S., & Backman, C. L. (2015). eHealth, participatory medicine, and ethical care: A focus group study of patients' and health care providers' use of health-related internet information. *Journal of Medical Internet Research, 17*(6), e155.

Triberti, S., & Chirico, A. (2017). Healthy avatars, healthy people: Care engagement through the shared experience of virtual worlds. In G. Graffigna (Ed.), *Transformative healthcare practice through patient engagement* (pp. 247–275). Hershey: IGI Global.

Triberti, S., Durosini, I., Aschieri, F., Villani, D., & Riva, G. (2017). Changing avatars, changing selves? The influence of social and contextual expectations on digital rendition of identity. *Cyberpsychology, Behavior and Social Networking, 20*(8), 501–507.

Triberti, S., Bigi, S., Rossi, M. G., Caretto, A., Laurenzi, A., Dozio, N., … Riva, G. (2018, January). The active ageing mobile app for diabetes self-management: First adherence data and analysis of patients' in-app notes. In *International symposium on pervasive computing paradigms for mental health* (pp. 129–138). Springer, Cham.

Triberti, S., Savioni, L., Sebri, V., & Pravettoni, G. (2019). eHealth for improving quality of life in breast cancer patients: A systematic review. *Cancer Treatment Reviews, 74*, 1–14.

Van der Krieke, L., Emerencia, A. C., Boonstra, N., Wunderink, L., de Jonge, P., & Sytema, S. (2013). A web-based tool to support shared decision making for people with a psychotic disorder: Randomized controlled trial and process evaluation. *Journal of Medical Internet Research, 15*(10), e216.

Van Dyck, D., Plaete, J., Cardon, G., Crombez, G., & De Bourdeaudhuij, I. (2016). Effectiveness of the self-regulation eHealth intervention 'MyPlan1. 0.'on physical activity levels of recently retired Belgian adults: a randomized controlled trial. *Health Education Research, 31*(5), 653–664.

Villani, D., Gatti, E., Triberti, S., Confalonieri, E., & Riva, G. (2016). Exploration of virtual body-representation in adolescence: The role of age and sex in avatar customization. *Springerplus, 5*(1), 740.

Vogenberg, F. R., Barash, C. I., & Pursel, M. (2010). Personalized medicine: Part 1: Evolution and development into theranostics. *Pharmacy and Therapeutics, 35*(10), 560.

Zhang, A., Sun, H., Wang, P., Han, Y., & Wang, X. (2012). Future perspectives of personalized medicine in traditional Chinese medicine: A systems biology approach. *Complementary Therapies in Medicine, 20*(1–2), 93–99.

Zitelli, A., & Palmer, R. (1979). Le teorie mediche sulla peste e il contesto veneziano. *AAVV, Venezia e la peste, 1348*(1797), 21–28.

Chapter 5
Predictive Precision Medicine: Towards the Computational Challenge

Cosimo Tuena, Michelle Semonella, Javier Fernández-Álvarez, Desirée Colombo, and Pietro Cipresso

1 Introduction

Medicine is an evolving field that updates its applications thanks to recent advances from a broad spectrum of sciences such as biology, chemistry, statistics, mathematics, engineering and life and social sciences. Generally, discoveries in such sciences are applied to medicine with three main aims of preventing, diagnosing and treating a wide range of medical conditions.

The current approach to diseases can be summarized with the "one-size-fits all" statement; although this view of medicine has been used for the past 30 years, applications of effective treatment, for example, can lack efficacy and have adverse or unpredictable reactions in individual patients (Roden 2016).

Precision medicine is the extension and the evolution of the current approach to patient's management (Ramaswami et al. 2018). Unlike "one-size-fits all" approach, precision medicine is mainly preventive and proactive rather than reactive (Mathur and Sutton 2017) (cfr. Chap. 3). Barak Obama, who claimed the importance of "delivering the right treatments, at the right time, every time to the right person", has highlighted the critical impact of this emerging initiative in healthcare practice.

C. Tuena · M. Semonella
Applied Technology for NeuroPsychology Lab, Istituto Auxologico Italiano, Milan, Italy

J. Fernández-Álvarez
Department of Psychology, Università Cattolica del Sacro Cuore, Milan, Italy

D. Colombo
Department of Basic Psychology, Clinic and Psychobiology, Universitat Jaume I, Castellón, Spain

P. Cipresso (✉)
Applied Technology for NeuroPsychology Lab, Istituto Auxologico Italiano, Milan, Italy

Department of Psychology, Università Cattolica del Sacro Cuore, Milan, Italy
e-mail: pietro.cipresso@unicatt.it

G. Pravettoni, S. Triberti (eds.), *P5 eHealth: An Agenda for the Health Technologies of the Future*, https://doi.org/10.1007/978-3-030-27994-3_5

The personalized approach has been therefore emerged as a critique to an oversimplified and reductive medicine to disease categorization and treatment. Precision medicine uses a broad spectrum of data, ranging from biological to social information, tailoring diagnosis, prognosis and therapy on patient's needs and characteristics, in accordance to the P5 approach.

Another crucial element of this initiative is the use of informatics: incorporating technology would allow to create a data ecosystem that merges biological information and clinical phenotypes, thanks to imaging, laboratory test and health records, in order to better identify and treat the disease affecting the individual, reducing financial and time efforts and improving the quality of life of the patients.

The present chapter will focus on the potential of predictive precision medicine as new approach to health sciences and clinical practice, giving an overview on the tools, the methodology and a concrete application of the P5 approach.

2 Predictive Medicine and Precision Medicine

Among healthcare applications, predictive medicine is a relatively new area, and it can be defined as the use of laboratory and genetic tests to predict either the onset of a disease in an individual or deterioration or amelioration of current disease, to estimate the risk for a certain outcome and predict which treatment will be the most effective on the individual (Jen and Teoli 2019; Jen and Varacallo 2019; Valet and Tárnok 2003). In this sense, biomarkers could be used to forecast disease onset, prognosis and therapy outcome. Biomarker or biological marker indicates a medical sign that can be measured in an objective way, accurately and reproducibly; the World Health Organization defined biomarker as "almost any measurement reflecting an interaction between a biological system and a potential hazard, which may be chemical, physical, or biological. The measured response may be functional and physiological, biochemical at the cellular level, or a molecular interaction" (Strimbu and Tavel 2010). Biomarkers are used for drug development and clinical outcome; if the current approach to clinical trials is "one-size-fits-all" (i.e. the effect of a treatment is similar for the whole sample), the future of medicine is to provide the "the right treatment for the right patient at the right time", identifying different subgroups depending on certain biomarkers that respond to an optimal therapy (Chen et al. 2015).

As we have seen in the previous chapters, precision medicine is one of the P5 approach's features that tailor healthcare applications on the basis of individual genes, environment and lifestyle (Hodson 2016). If personalized medicine takes into account patient's genes but also beliefs, preferences and social context, precision medicine is a model heavily based on data, analytics and information; thus, the latter approach has a wide "ecosystem" that includes patients, clinicians, researchers, technologies, genomics and data sharing (Ginsburg and Phillips 2018). In order to realize precision medicine, it is crucial to determine biomarkers using either omic (i.e. genomic, proteomic, epigenetic and so on) data alone or in combination with environmental and lifestyle information (Wang et al. 2017) with the objective of creating prognostic, diagnostic and therapeutic interventions based on patient's needs (Mirnezami et al. 2012).

This new concept of medicine involves the medical institutions that collect every day healthcare information, such as biomedical images or signals. New analytical methods computed by computer, such as machine learning, prompted the "Big Data Revolution"; thus Big Data analysis in predictive medicine (Jen and Teoli 2019; Jen and Varacallo 2019), computational psychometrics (Cipresso 2015; Cipresso et al. 2015; von Davier 2017) and precision medicine (Richard Leff and Yang 2015) may soon benefit from huge amount of medical information and computational techniques (Cipresso and Immekus 2017). New technologies such as virtual reality enable to extract online quantitative and computational data for each individual to deepen the study of cognitive processes (Cipresso 2015; Muratore et al. 2019; Tuena et al. 2019). eHealth generally is an accurate instrument in collecting data; furthermore, Big Data differ from conventional analyses in three ways according to Mayer-Schönberger and Ingelsson (Mayer-Schönberger and Ingelsson 2018): data of the phenomenon under question are extracted in a comprehensive manner; machine learning such as neural networks are preferred for statistical analyses compared to conventional methods; and finally, Big Data do not only answer to questions but generate new hypotheses.

Consequently, technologies and informatics will gradually become the future of medicine (Regierer et al. 2013). eHealth aims at using biomedical data for scientific questions, decision-making (cfr. Chap. 4) and problem-solving (Jen and Teoli 2019; Jen and Varacallo 2019) in accordance with the P5 approach. On the one hand, informatics is crucial for precision medicine since it manages Big Data, creates learning systems, gives access for individual involvement and supports precision intervention from translational research (Frey et al. 2016); on the other hand, clinical informatics is crucial for predictive medicine providing clinicians tools that able to give information about individual at risk, disease onset and how to intervene (Jen and Teoli 2019; Jen and Varacallo 2019). The importance of informatics in the field of medicine is confirmed by the fact that in the United States the use of electronic health records grew from 11.8% to 39.6% among physicians from 2007 to 2012 (Hsiao et al. 2014).

Besides the medical and scientific elements of precision medicine, this field has an impact also on patient and global population (Ginsburg and Phillips 2018; Pritchard et al. 2017). In particular, the precision medicine coalition's healthcare working group defined novel challenges within this field:

- **Education and awareness**: Precision medicine is complex and sometimes confusing; awareness should be improved in potential consumers and healthcare providers, and education within the scientific and clinic areas should integrate the precision medicine approach.
- **Patient empowerment**: Precision medicine is a way to engage and empower the patient. However, consent form needs to clarify the use of molecular information, and providers do not properly involve patient in healthcare decision-making,

and preferences are not always taken into account; lastly, privacy and security of the digital data must be improved and assured.

- **Value recognition**: There are ambivalent sentiments concerning precision medicine, where stakeholders think that precision medicine can be beneficial for patients and healthcare system, whereas payers and providers are not sure to modify policies and practices without clear positive evidence of clinical and economic value.
- **Infrastructure and information management**: In order to pursue, the precision medicine approach is needed to effectively manage the massive amount of data and the connections among the infrastructures; for instance, processes and policies should assure clear communications across healthcare providers, genetic patients' data could be gathered with clinical information within electronic health records, and medical data need to be standardized across platforms.
- **Ensuring access to care**: This point needs a shift in the perspective of stakeholders that is achieved by covering the aforementioned key points; at the moment, insurance companies do not cover high-quality diagnostic procedures, electronic health records should be upgraded to integrate complex biological data, some physicians avoid to embrace the precision medicine approach due to misleading perception (e.g. cost/benefit distortions), there is no guideline that coordinates the partners and products, and services cannot be used by population especially in rural environments.

Predictive precision medicine in the P5 approach can be defined as the merging of these two new fields of medical sciences by means of biomarkers to forecast disease onset, progression and its treatment tailored on individual features like omic, environmental and lifestyle elements that could lead to significant improvement from patients' life to global population and healthcare systems.

3 Imaging Techniques, Artificial Intelligence and Machine Learning

3.1 Imaging Techniques

In the context of predictive medicine and precision medicine, biomedical imaging instruments used in radiology are the most promising techniques and methods (Herold et al. 2016; Jen and Teoli 2019; Jen and Varacallo 2019). In particular, with radiology techniques, it is possible to extract structural, functional and metabolic information that can be used for diagnostic, prognostic and therapeutic purposes (Herold et al. 2016). Imaging techniques (Jen and Varacallo 2019) acquire a vital role not only in applied medicine but also in system biology that attempts to model the structure and the dynamics of complex biological systems (Kherlopian et al.

2008). Model imaging techniques enable to visualize multidimensional and multiparametrical data, such as concentration, tissue characteristics, surfaces and also temporal information (Eils and Athale 2003). According to Kherlopian and colleagues (Kherlopian et al. 2008), the most promising imaging instruments will be microscopy methods, ultrasound, computed tomography (CT), magnetic resonance imaging (MRI) and positron emission tomography (PET); advances in biomedical engineering will improve spatial and temporal resolution of such images, but with the introduction of contrast agents and molecular probes, biomedical images will allow for the visualization of anatomical structures, cells and molecular dynamics, and consequently, microCT, microMRI and microPET are going to be at the centre of basic and applied research.

Multiphoton microscopy, atomic force microscopy and electron microscopy are capable of giving, respectively, cell structure, cell surface and protein structure with a spatial resolution of nanometres; enabling ultrasound had a great impact in cardiology, where, for instance, computer is used to interpret echo waveforms bouncing back from tissue and create images of the vascular system with a resolution of micrometres. CT by means of intrinsic differences in X-ray absorption provided imaging with a high spatial resolution (12–50 μm), that is, lung or bone imaging. Interestingly, microCT in combination with volumetric decomposition allows to represent bone microarchitecture. MRI, thanks to the use of strong magnetic field, creates anatomical images with a good spatial resolution; if MRI is combined with magnetic resonance spectroscopy, it can provide anatomical and biochemical information of a particular region of the organ; if one's interest is functional activation of the brain, then functional MRI detects differences in oxygenated and deoxygenated haemoglobin that lead to a change in contrast of the image. MicroMRI is used in animal studies at the moment and uses higher magnetic field compared to MRI; with such technique, it is possible to track stem cells, monitor the proliferation of immune cells and follow embryological development. In PET radioactive tracers, the most used is fluorodeoxyglucose (FDG), which is incorporated in molecules to provide metabolic information and therapeutic effects on the disease as well. Even if it is possible to study a specific metabolic activity of interest, the spatial resolution (1–2 mm) is lower compared to the aforementioned techniques; however, microPET has a spatial volumetric of 8 mm^3, with incoming scanners having higher resolution and bigger field of view.

The use of imaging tools such as CT, MRI and PET is growing increasingly, for instance, in the United States from 1996 to 2010 in six healthcare systems, the usage increased by, respectively, 7.8%, 10% and 57% (Smith-Bindman et al. 2012). However, imaging techniques are several in the present chapter; we only focused on the main technologies used in medical field and in particular radiology. This underlines the importance of technology and eHealth as opportunity for improving precision medicine at large.

3.2 Artificial Intelligence and Machine Learning

Artificial intelligence (AI) aims at simulating human cognition (Hassabis et al. 2017). One of the recent technologies used within the context of AI is machine learning (ML); ML enables machine to have a human-like intelligence without prior programming (Das et al. 2015). Moreover, ML is the most used method to analyse data and make prediction using models and algorithms (Angra and Ahuja 2017). Within the context of ML, deep learning (DL) and neural network (NN) assume great relevance (Ker et al. 2018; Schmidhuber 2015). The concept of NN was first introduced in 1943 by McCulloch and Pitts and found its application in the Rosenblat's Perceptron; an artificial NN consists of a layer of neurons that links inputs that perceive a certain stimuli, hidden neurons that get activated via weighted connections of active neurons and output that gives the computation made by the NN. DL is multiple layers of artificial neural networks, wherein the machine can learn details and merge them in high-level features in brain-like manner. DL and NN enabled complex computations using supervised, unsupervised and reinforcement learning. The algorithms used in ML can be classified as follows (Das et al. 2015; Hassabis et al. 2017; Jiang et al. 2017):

- **Supervised learning**: When a comparison between output and expected output is made, then error is computed and adjusted to give the wanted output; within the context of supervised learning, the most used DL algorithm is convolutional neural network (CNN), especially used in image recognition and visual learning in 2D and 3D images, enabling the analyses of X-ray and CT or MRI images; recurrent neural network (RNN) is used for text analysis task (e.g. machine translation, text prediction, image caption) similar to a working memory function and evolved into the long- and short -term memory networks to avoid vanishing gradient problem; indeed, an application of AI in this field is a natural language processing that can be used for extracting medical notes and connecting these to medical data. Other supervised learning methods are linear regression, logistic regression, naïve Bayes, decision tree, nearest neighbour, random forest, discriminant analysis, support vector machine (SVM) and NN.
- **Unsupervised learning**: In this case, the machine discovers and adjusts itself based on input. For example, an autoencoder input codes the stimuli-gathered codings and reconstructs from these the output; in this case, the output must be as close as possible to the input information; restricted Boltzmann machines are composed of visible and hidden layers that reconstruct the input estimating the probability distribution of the original input; in deep belief network, the output of a restricted Boltzmann machine is the input of another Boltzmann machine; finally, generative adversarial networks are generative models that are composed of two competing CNNs: the first CNN generates artificial training images, and the second CNN discriminates real training images from artificial ones; the desired expectation is that the discriminator cannot tell the difference between the two images; this algorithm is very promising for medical image analyses; other unsupervised methods are clustering, which can be used to divide data in

groups, and principal component analysis that reduces data dimension without losing critical information and then creating groups.

- **Reinforcement learning**: In this case, learning is enhanced with a reward when the machine executes a "winning" choice; similarly, Q-learning algorithm (Rodrigues et al. 2008) allows to compute the future rewards when the machine is performing a certain action in a particular state in order to keep on acting in an optimal manner.
- **Recommender system**: In this case, the online user customizes a site as what happens in e-commerce.

ML problems include pattern classification, regression, control, system identification and prediction that can be summarized into two main elements: developing algorithms that quantify relations among data and using these to make prediction on new data (Wernick et al. 2014).

3.3 Medical Imaging and Machine Learning

ML and AI find in medical imaging field a concrete application in order to analyse images and help physician with particular regard in the field of radiology in decision-making processes improving patient's management (Jiang et al. 2017; Ker et al. 2018; Kim et al. 2018). Indeed, the P5 approach underlines the importance of decision-making process and the usage of eHealth in order to improve it. ML technology is used in the sector of medical imaging for computer-aided diagnosis (CADx) and computer-aided detection (CADe); the former can also help to identify region properties useful for surgery. In radiology, CADx and CADe usages are, respectively, classification and detection although ML techniques can be used for anatomy educational purposes (i.e. localization) and to facilitate surgery (i.e. segmentation, registration) (Kim et al. 2018).

According to the review conducted on PubMed from 2013 to 2016 by Jiang and co-authors (Jiang et al. 2017), AI applications critical in medical field are cardiology, cancer and neurology. In their report, Jiang and colleagues evidenced that the fields of medical application of AI are diagnostic imaging, genetic and electrodiagnosis, with diagnostic imaging showing the greater impact on research. As concerns the disease conditions, the order of impact on research activity are neoplasms, nervous system, cardiovascular, urogenital, pregnancy, digestive, respiratory, skin, endocrine and nutritional; finally, the most used algorithms in this field are NN and SVM, and in particular, DL technology is applied mostly in diagnostic imaging and electrodiagnosis; interestingly, from 2013 to 2016 CNN increased the application in literature, whereas RNN diminished, and deep belief network and deep neural network remained stable across the periods.

In particular, CNN, autoencoders and RNN are excellent algorithms for medical imaging analysis (Kim et al. 2018). Convolution that is based on addition and multiplication is suitable for image recognition; the procedure takes into account connected information (i.e. voxel or pixel); within convolution layers, there are pooling layers that increase the field of view, and then fully connected layers activate previous layers; autoencoders are composed of multiple perceptrons; encoders can be stacked and can be used to de-noise image of input data; and finally RNN uses feedback and current data enabling to model sequential data with spatial and temporal information. CNN architectures can be used to detect different organ (e.g. brain, liver, heart, prostate or retina) lesions or diseases; to predict disease course, treatment response and survival; and to classify disease, lesion and cell using CT, MRI, PET and other imaging techniques (e.g. retina image, mammography or fluorescent image). Autoencoders have been used in research to detect lesion with breast histology images, predict risk for cognitive deficits and classify lung and breast lesions, whereas stacked autoencoders have been applied for segmentation and image enhancement/generation. Also other algorithms are applied in radiology, for instance, reinforcement learning in combination with data mining helps in decision-making for physicians in cancer diagnosis, for segmentation tasks and for classification of lung nodules (Rodrigues et al. 2008). A critical element of these technologies is that before applying AI to medical imaging and more broadly to healthcare system, algorithms need to be trained with data derived from clinical activities and in different forms; for example, 1.2 million of training data are being used to teach DL algorithms on MRI brain imaging; by the way, the quality of DL techniques depends on the quality of training data; this issue can be improved by adopting multisite, standardized and methodologically adequate acquisition protocols (Jiang et al. 2017).

4 Predictive Precision Medicine in Neurodegenerative Diseases

An increasing lifespan and expectancy with a reduction of mortality result in an increment in aged population in our society; consequently, these factors have brought the attention of scientific and clinical community to chronic age-related or degenerative diseases. Due to the complexity of the aetiology and pathogenesis, resulting in interplay among genetic, epigenetic and environment, prevention (primary, secondary and tertiary) (cfr. Chap. 3) and, in particular, predictive and precision medicine assume a crucial role as features of the P5 approach, with omic approach to biology and computational methods acquiring a relevant position (Licastro and Caruso 2010; Reitz 2016). In particular, predictive genetic testing and molecular genetic diagnosis have well-established position in clinical practice and translational research in the field of neurodegenerative disorders (Paulsen et al. 2013). Indeed, neurodegenerative diseases have specific gene profiles (Bertram and Tanzi 2005). For instance, symptomatic testing in Alzheimer's disease (AD) requires neurological and neuropsychological examination; then genetic counselling and risk administration are determined: either an autosomal dominant history is present or the onset is early or sporadic, or there is a nonautosomal dominant family clustering; in the first case, genetic testing is offered; if not or in the second case, it is possible to discuss availability of genetic research and/or DNA banking; always in the first case, post-test results are emitted and follow-up/predictive testing for relative is provided; conversely for predictive testing, family mutation in relevant genes (PSEN1, PSEN2 or APP) is known; genetic and risk counselling is provided; neurological, neuropsychological and psychiatric evaluations are offered; and then genetic test and follow-up follow the latter step (Goldman et al. 2011).

Neurological disorders account for 17% of global deaths, and precision medicine gathering genomics, electronic medical records and stem cell models might be vital for therapeutic interventions in neurology; in this sense, drugs tap common symptoms, but adopting a precision medicine approach, it is useful to create drugs that target group of people with similar genetic variation (Gibbs et al. 2018). Besides drug administration, precision medicine can be applied in the context of neurodegenerative diseases to evaluate preclinical stages, facilitate differential diagnosis and define the better treatment at the right moment taking into account genes, epigenetic modifiers and nongenetic factors on neurodegeneration; the combination of these elements should be used to create a patient's omic profile (Strafella et al. 2018).

4.1 Current Application: From Dementias to Parkinson's Disease

As already mentioned, ML approaches could be very useful in the field of brain imaging for classification and preventive aims. We will provide some interesting studies of ML within the context of preventive precision medicine for neurodegenerative disorders in order to highlight the importance of technology, and eHealth specifically, into precision medicine.

Katako and colleagues (Katako et al. 2018) used well-known FDG-PET metabolic biomarker (Dubois et al. 2007) from images from four datasets of the Alzheimer's disease neuroimaging initiative. The researchers compared five machine-based classification (i.e. voxel-wise general linear model, subprofile modelling and SVM). Subprofile modelling is a type of PCA used for differential diagnosis and prognosis in neurodegeneration, whereas SVM is a form of supervised learning used to solve binary classification. Subprofile modelling was utilized with two PCA approaches (single principal component and linear combination of principal components); for SVM iterative single-data algorithm or sequential minimal optimization was applied. All five methods discriminated patients and controls, when compared with tenfold cross-validation SVA with iterative single-data algorithm gave the best results in terms of sensitivity (0.84) and specificity (0.95). In terms of prediction of AD from mild cognitive impairment (MCI), this SVA algorithm had the best performance; interestingly, when comparing PET and single-photon emission computed tomography (SPECT), the iterative single-data algorithm showed higher sensitivity compared to sequential minimal optimization SVM, whereas the latter has higher specificity compared to the former. To test clinical application of the method, a retrospective imaging study was conducted with MCI and subjective cognitive complaints individuals referred from the local memory clinic. All five methods classified as AD the majority of patients later diagnosed with this disease; however, patients who later developed dementia with Lewy body (DLB) and Parkinson's disease dementia (PDD) were diagnosed as having AD, showing nonspecificity for different types of dementias. Despite that, FDG-PET images showed that DLB and PDD brain pathology suggest AD-like biomarker that is not present in non-demented Parkinson's diseases (PDND) individuals when using SVM algorithms. Lama and co-authors (Lama et al. 2017) classified structural images from the Alzheimer's disease neuroimaging initiative. Using structural MRI (i.e. grey matter tissue volume), the researchers compared brain images from patients with AD, MCI and healthy controls using SVM, import vector machine (IVM) based on kernel logistic regression and regularized extreme machine learning (RELM); moreover, to reduce the dimensionality of data, PCA was performed, and permutation testing such as 70/30 cross-validation, tenfold cross-validation and leave-one-out cross-validation was applied. The best classifiers appeared to be the RELM with PCA for feature selection approach; this machine improved classification of AD from MCI and controls. In particular, binary classification (AD vs. controls) with PCA revealed that in terms of accuracy, there was no significant difference, but RELM is better than others with tenfold cross-validation, whereas SVM is better than the latter with leave-one-out cross-validation. Sensitivity was 77.51% for SVM, and specificity was 90.63% for RELM with tenfold cross-validation, whereas with leave-one-out cross-validation, IVM has a sensitivity of 87.10% and RELM a specificity of 83.54%. Multiclass classification (AD vs. MCI vs. controls) with PCA showed that RELM with tenfold and leave-one-out cross-validation has an accuracy of 59.81% and 61.58% and a specificity of 62.25%. Another study that used MRI is the one of Donnelly-Kehoe et al. (Donnelly-Kehoe et al. 2018). In their research, neuromorphometric features from MRI classify controls, MCI, MCI converted to AD and AD. Participants were divided in three groups according to Mini-Mental State Examination (MMSE) scores with the aim of searching the main morphologic features; these were used to design a multiclassifier system (MCS) composed of three subclassifiers trained on data selected depending on MMSE; MCS was compared with three classification algorithms: random forest, SVM and Ada-Boost. MCS with three architectures each outperformed single classifiers in terms of accuracy, and for area under the receiver operating curve (AUC), multiclass AUC was 0.83 for controls, 0.76 for MCI converted to AD, 0.65 for MCI and 0.95 for AD. Accuracy for neurodegenerative detection (AD + MCI converted to AD) was 81%. Random forest and SVM had similar performances, but the former was chosen as the best algorithm since it has few parameters. In particular, accuracy on neurodegenerative detection for the three random forests was 0.71, 0.63 and 0.81. The authors claim that MCS based on cognitive scoring can help MRI AD diagnosis compared to well-established algorithms. Interestingly, Guo and colleagues (Guo et al. 2017) developed an ML technology that exploits hypernetwork able to overcome conventional network methods and fMRI data of AD individuals. After data acquisition, they built the hypernetwork's connectivity and extracted brain regions with a nonparametric test method and subgraph features with frequently scoring feature selection algorithm; then, kernel (vector and graph, respectively) matrix classification with multikernel SVM was computed. Findings from brain regions and graph features are in line with previous network disruption in AD (Buckner et al. 2008). SVM classification was used for classification of the sample (AD, early MCI and late MCI), and the hypernetwork enabled to extract interactions and topological information. The results of the ML were compared with conventional methods based on partial and Pearson correlations. Findings reveal that the method identifies both interactive and representative high-order information; moreover, AUC for brain region features was 0.831 and 0.762 for graph features but for multifeature classification was 0.919. Multifeature classification can therefore ameliorate AD diagnosis based on biomarker.

Interestingly, ML can be used also to compute electroencephalography (EEG) biomarker in order to identify AD pathology and drug intervention (Simpraga et al. 2017). Data were used to calculate muscarinic acetylcholine receptor antagonist (mAChR) index in healthy participants who received scopolamine to simulate cognitive deficits from 14 EEG biomarkers (spatial and temporal biomarker algorithm); the index had cross-validated accuracy, sensitivity, specificity and precision ranging from 88% to 92% in classifying performances compared to single biomarkers. The mAChR index successfully classified AD patients with accuracy of 62%, 35% sensitivity, 91% specificity and 81% precision; also an AD index was computed from 12 EEG biomarker with accuracy, sensitivity, specificity and precision ranging from 87% to 97%. The findings are useful not only for diagnosis between healthy participants and patients with AD but also for experimental pharmacology because the index assesses the well-known AD cholinergic electrophysiology and drug penetration in this disease.

Frontotemporal dementia (FTD) is one of the most common causes of early onset dementia; among FTD profiles, behavioural FTD is the most frequent and is characterized by specific biomarker (Piguet et al. 2011). Meyer and co-authors used MRI from multicentre cohort to predict diagnosis in each single patient showing the potential of precision medicine (Meyer et al. 2017). They calculated brain atrophy differences between controls and patients and used SVM to differentiate these groups on an individual level. Grey matter density from the conjunction analyses of the cohorts evidenced an overlap in the frontal poles bilaterally. When using the algorithm to predict diagnosis individually, accuracy ranged from 71.1% to 78.9% in the same centre sample (19 behavioural FTD patients vs. 19 controls) and from 78.8% to 84.6% in the whole sample analyses (52 behavioural FTD patients vs. 52 controls). The better predictive region was the frontal lobe compared to the temporal area (80.7% vs. 78.8%); the accuracy increased when accuracy was computed for frontal and temporal regions together and furthermore ameliorated when adding other relevant brain regions such as insula and basal ganglia. Despite researchers found an intercentre variability, they encourage the use of ML and imaging techniques for predictive purposes based on biomarker for personalized early detection of brain degeneration.

Another neurodegenerative disease that represents a social burden is Parkinson's disease (PD). Biomarkers and imaging can improve the diagnosis of neurodegenerative diseases such as PD (Pievani et al. 2011). Abós and co-authors used ML to define biomarker associated with cognitive status in PD individuals (Abós et al. 2017). Functional connectivity was used to assess PD depending on cognitive profile (with MCI or without MCI) with ML methods and resting-state fMRI. In their study, supervised SVM algorithm, functional connectomics data, neuropsychological profile, leave-one-out cross-validation and independent sample (training group vs. validation group) validation for the model were applied. Leave-one-out cross-validation for subject classification prediction for PD-MCI and PD-nonMCI was for both 82.6%; the independent sample validation correctly classified with the trained SVM machine the participants with AUC of 0.81. Leave-one-out cross-validation and randomized logistic regression were used to select the most relevant edges (21) and nodes (34) of the network. There was an alteration of the edges for the PD-MCI compared to PD-nonMCI group. For 16 edges, connectivity was reduced in the former group, for 13 of these edges, connectivity was impaired also compared to controls, but for the remaining 5, the network was stronger in PD-MCI compared to PD-nonMCI. For the 16 weakened edges, correlations were found with executive functions, visuospatial deficits, levadopa daily dosage and disease duration. This methodology proposed by the authors shows that ML and fMRI could be useful for PD cognitive diagnosis and assessment.

ML can successfully be applied also to nonimaging data to predict the risk for dementia from population-based surveys (de Langavant et al. 2018). Langavant and colleagues developed unsupervised ML classification with PCA and hierarchical clustering on the Health and Retirement Study (HRS; 2002–2003, N = 18,165 individuals) and validated the algorithm in the Survey of Health, Ageing and Retirement in Europe (SHARE; 2010–2012, N = 58,202 individuals). The accuracy of this method was assessed with a subgroup of the HRS with dementia diagnosis from previous study. The machine identified three clusters from HRS: individuals with no functional and motor (e.g. walking) impairment, with motor impairment only and with both functional and motor deficits. The latter group showed a high likelihood for dementia (probability of dementia >0.95; area under the curve [AUC] = 0.91) also when removing cognitive/behavioural measures. Similar clusters were found in SHARE. After 3.9 years follow-up, survival rate for HRS and SHARE in cluster 3 were 39.2% and 62.2%; surviving participants in this cluster showed functional and motor impairments over the same period. The authors claim that the algorithm is able to classify people at risk for dementia and survival and therefore use this classification for prevention and trial assignment.

In their review, Dallora and colleagues (Dallora et al. 2017) found that for the prognosis of dementia, the most applied ML technique is SVM; among ML, neuroimaging studies (i.e. MRI and PET) were most frequent compared to cognitive/

behavioural, genetic, lab tests and demographic data with the main of predicating the proportion of MCI individuals that will develop AD. The researchers in terms of validation procedure, datasets used, number or records within the same dataset and follow-up period found limitations. However, defining biomarkers in the field of neurodegenerative diseases could improve diagnosis and treatment and consolidate the role of precision medicine and prediction of disease progress (Dallora et al. 2017; Reitz 2016; Rosenberg 2017). As we have seen, technologies (and eHealth especially) could be a good instrument, also in the context of the P5 approach and future medicine.

5 Conclusion

In this chapter, we elucidated the potential role of predictive precision medicine as a feature of the P5 approach with a particular focus on radiological imaging and ML algorithms applied in neurology. Despite the benefits of precision medicine, the complexity of this approach could be simplified with artificial intelligence methods that can reduce the amount of information and target specific biomarker useful for diagnosis, prognosis and treatment. We reported excellent evidences that this approach could improve the management of neurodegenerative disorders (i.e. AD, PD, FTD, MCI, DLB, PDD) from different perspectives: individual and whole sample and metabolic, structural, functional, electrophysiological and cognitive/behavioural methods. For this reason, we encourage the healthcare system that in this sense comprises of researchers, clinicians, institutions, providers and stakeholders to embrace this vision of medicine.

References

Abós, A., Baggio, H. C., Segura, B., García-díaz, A. I., Compta, Y., Martí, M. J., … Junqué, C. (2017). Discriminating cognitive status in Parkinson's disease through functional connectomics and machine learning. *Scientific Reports, 7*(45347). https://doi.org/10.1038/srep45347.

Angra, S., & Ahuja, S. (2017). Machine learning and its applications: A review. In *Machine learning and its applications: A review* (pp. 57–60).

Bertram, L., & Tanzi, R. E. (2005). The genetic epidemiology of neurodegenerative disease. *The Journal of Clinical Investigation, 115*(6), 1449–1457.

Buckner, R. L., Andrews-Hanna, J. R., & Schacter, D. L. (2008). The brain's default network: Anatomy, function, and relevance to disease. *Annals of the New York Academy of Sciences, 1124*, 1–38. https://doi.org/10.1196/annals.1440.011.

Chen, J. J., Lu, T. P., Chen, Y. C., & Lin, W. J. (2015). Predictive biomarkers for treatment selection: Statistical considerations. *Biomarkers in Medicine, 9*(11), 1121–1135.

Cipresso, P. (2015). Modeling behavior dynamics using computational psychometrics within virtual worlds. *Frontiers in Psychology, 6*, 1725.

Cipresso, P., & Immekus, J. C. (2017). Back to the future of quantitative psychology and measurement: Psychometrics in the twenty-first century. *Frontiers in Psychology, 8*, 2099.

Cipresso, P., Matic, A., Giakoumis, D., & Ostrovsky, Y. (2015). Advances in computational psychometrics. *Computational and Mathematical Methods in Medicine, 2015*, 1.

Dallora, A. L., Eivazzadeh, S., Mendes, E., Berglund, J., & Anderberg, P. (2017). Machine learning and microsimulation techniques on the prognosis of dementia : A systematic literature review. *PLoS One, 12*(6), e0179804.

Das, S., Dey, A., Pal, A., & Roy, N. (2015). Applications of artificial intelligence in machine learning : Review and Prospect. *International Journal of Computer Applications, 115*(9), 31–41.

de Langavant, L. C., Bayen, E., & Yaffe, K. (2018). Unsupervised machine learning to identify high likelihood of dementia in population-based surveys: Development and validation study. *Journal of Medical Internet Research, 20*(7), e10493.

Donnelly-Kehoe, P. A., Pascariello, G. O., & Gomez, J. C. (2018). Looking for Alzheimer's disease morphometric signatures using machine learning techniques. *Journal of Neuroscience Methods, 15*(302), 24–34. https://doi.org/10.1016/j.jneumeth.2017.11.013.

Dubois, B., Feldman, H. H., Jacova, C., DeKosky, S. T., Barberger-Gateau, P., Cummings, J., … Scheltens, P. (2007). Research criteria for the diagnosis of Alzheimer's disease: Revising the NINCDS-ADRDA criteria. *Lancet Neurology, 6*(8), 734–746. https://doi.org/10.1016/S1474-4422(07)70178-3.

Eils, R., & Athale, C. (2003). Computational imaging in cell biology. *Journal of Cell Biology, 161*(3), 477–481.

Frey, L. J., Bernstam, E. V., & Denny, J. C. (2016). Precision medicine informatics. *Journal of the American Medical Informatics Association, 23*(4), 668–670.

Gibbs, R. M., Lipnick, S., Bateman, J. W., Chen, L., Cousins, H. C., Hubbard, E. G., … Rubin, L. L. (2018). Forum toward precision medicine for neurological and neuropsychiatric disorders. *Cell Stem Cell, 23*(5), 21. https://doi.org/10.1016/j.stem.2018.05.019.

Ginsburg, G. S., & Phillips, K. A. (2018). Precision medicine : From science to value. *Health Affairs, 37*(5), 694–701. https://doi.org/10.1377/hlthaff.2017.1624.Precision.

Goldman, J. S., Hahn, S. E., Catania, J. W., Larusse-Eckert, S., Butson, M. B., Rumbaugh, M., … Bird, T. (2011). Genetic counseling and testing for Alzheimer disease: Joint practice guidelines of the American College of Medical Genetics and the National Society of Genetic Counselors. *Genetics in Medicine, 13*(6), 597.

Guo, H., Zhang, F., Chen, J., Xu, Y., & Xiang, J. (2017). Machine learning classification combining multiple features of a hyper-network of fMRI data in Alzheimer's disease. *Frontiers in Neuroscience, 11*(615). https://doi.org/10.3389/fnins.2017.00615.

Hassabis, D., Kumaran, D., Summerfield, C., & Botvinick, M. (2017). Neuroscience-Inspired Artificial Intelligence. *Neuron, 95*(2), 245–258. https://doi.org/10.1016/j.neuron.2017.06.011.

Herold, C. J., Lewin, J. S., Wibmer, A. G., Thrall, J. H., Dixon, A. K., Schoenberg, S. O., … Muellner, A. (2016). Imaging in the age of precision medicine : Summary of the proceedings of the 10th biannual symposium of the International Society for Strategic Studies in Radiology. *Radiology, 279*(1), 226–238.

Hodson, R. (2016). Precision medicine. *Nature, 537*(7619), S49.

Hsiao, C.-J., Hing, E., & Ashman, J. (2014). Trendsinelectronichealthrecord system use among office-based physicians: United States, 2007–2012. *National Health Statistics Report, 75*, 1–18.

Jen, M.Y. & Teoli, D. Informatics. (2019 Jul 29. In: *StatPearls [Internet]*. Treasure Island (FL): StatPearls Publishing; 2019 Jan-. Available from: https://www.europepmc.org/books/NBK470564

Jen, M.Y. & Varacallo, M. Predictive Medicine. (2019 Jul 30). In: *StatPearls [Internet]*. Treasure Island (FL): StatPearls Publishing; 2019 Jan-. Available from: https://www.ncbi.nlm.nih.gov/books/NBK441941/

Jiang, F., Jiang, Y., Zhi, H., Dong, Y., Li, H., Ma, S., … Wang, Y. (2017). Artificial intelligence in healthcare: Past, present and future. *Stroke and Vascular Neurology, 2*(4), 230–243. https://doi.org/10.1136/svn-2017-000101.

Katako, A., Shelton, P., Goertzen, A. L., Levin, D., Bybel, B., Aljuaid, M., … Ko, J. H. (2018). Alzheimer's disease-related FDG- PET pattern which is also expressed in Lewy body dementia and Parkinson's disease dementia. *Scientific Reports, 8*(13236), 13236. https://doi.org/10.1038/s41598-018-31653-6.

Ker, J., Lipo, W., Rao, J., & Lim, T. (2018). Deep learning applications in medical image analysis. *IEEE Access, 6*, 9375–9389.

Kherlopian, A. R., Song, T., Duan, Q., Neimark, M. A., Po, M. J., Gohagan, J. K., & Laine, A. F. (2008). A review of imaging techniques for systems biology. *BMC Systems Biology, 2*(74), 74. https://doi.org/10.1186/1752-0509-2-74.

Kim, J., Hong, J., & Park, H. (2018). Prospects of deep learning for medical imaging. *Precision and Future Medicine, 2*(2), 37–52.

Lama, R. K., Gwak, J., Park, J., & Lee, S. (2017). Diagnosis of Alzheimer's disease based on structural MRI images using a regularized extreme learning machine and PCA features. *Journal of Healthcare Engineering, 2017*(5485080), 1.

Licastro, F., & Caruso, C. (2010). Predictive diagnostics and personalized medicine for the prevention of chronic degenerative diseases. *Immunity & Ageing, 7*(Suppl 1), S1. https://doi.org/10.1186/1742-4933-7-S1-S1.

Mathur, S., & Sutton, J. (2017). Personalized medicine could transform healthcare. *Journal of Biomedical Reports, 7*, 3–5. https://doi.org/10.3892/br.2017.922.

Mayer-Schönberger, V., & Ingelsson, E. (2018). Big data and medicine: A big deal? *Journal of Internal Medicine, 283*(5), 418–429.

Meyer, S., Mueller, K., Stuke, K., Bisenius, S., Diehl-schmid, J., Jessen, F., … Group FS. (2017). Predicting behavioral variant frontotemporal dementia with pattern classi fi cation in multicenter structural MRI data. *NeuroImage: Clinical, 14*, 656–662. https://doi.org/10.1016/j.nicl.2017.02.001.

Mirnezami, R., Nicholson, J., & Darzi, A. (2012). Preparing for precision medicine. *New England Journal of Medicine, 366*(6), 489–491.

Muratore, M., Tuena, C., Pedroli, E., Cipresso, P., & Riva, G. (2019). Virtual reality as a possible tool for the assessment of self-awareness. *Frontiers in Behavioural Neuroscience, 13*, 62.

Paulsen, J. S., Nance, M., Kim, J., Carlozzi, N. E., Panegyres, P. K., Erwin, C., … Williams, J. K. (2013). Progress in neurobiology a review of quality of life after predictive testing for and earlier identification of neurodegenerative diseases. *Progress in Neurobiology, 110*, 2–28. https://doi.org/10.1016/j.pneurobio.2013.08.003.

Pievani, M., De Haan, W., Wu, T., Seeley, W. W., Frisoni, G. B., & Giovanni, S. (2011). Functional network disruption in the degenerative dementias. *The Lancet Neurology, 10*(9), 829–843. https://doi.org/10.1016/S1474-4422(11)70158-2.

Piguet, O., Hornberger, M., Mioshi, E., & Hodges, J. R. (2011). Behavioural-variant frontotemporal dementia : Diagnosis, clinical staging, and management. *The Lancet Neurology, 10*(2), 162–172. https://doi.org/10.1016/S1474-4422(10)70299-4.

Pritchard, D. E., Moeckel, F., Villa, M. S., Housman, L. T., McCarty, C. A., & McLeod, H. L. (2017). Strategies for integrating personalized medicine into healthcare practice. *Personalized Medicine, 14*(2), 141–152.

Ramaswami, R., Bayer, R., & Galea, S. (2018). Precision medicine from a public health perspective. *Annual Review of Public Health, 39*(1.1), 1–16.

Regierer, B., Zazzu, V., Sudbrak, R., Kühn, A., & Lehrach, H. (2013). Future of medicine: Models in predictive diagnostics and personalized medicine. *Advances in Biochemical, Engeneering/Biotechnology, 133*, 15–33.

Reitz, C. (2016). Toward precision medicine in Alzheimer's disease. *Annals of Transaltional Medicine, 4*(6), 107. https://doi.org/10.21037/atm.2016.03.05.

Richard Leff, D., & Yang, G.-Z. (2015). Big data for precision medicine. *Engineering, 1*(3), 277–279.

Roden, D. M. (2016). Cardiovascular pharmacogenomics: Current status and future directions. *Journal of Human Genetics, 61*(1), 79. https://doi.org/10.1038/jhg.2015.78.Cardiovascular.

Rodrigues, V., Leite, C., Silva, A., & Paiva, A. (2008). *Application on reinforcement learning for diagnosis based on medical image*. (M. E. and N. M. M. Cornelius Weber, Ed.). IntechOpen. https://doi.org/10.5772/5291.

Rosenberg, G. A. (2017). Binswanger's disease: Biomarkers in the inflammatory form of vascular cognitive impairment and dementia. *Journal of Neurochemistry, 144*(5), 634–643. https://doi.org/10.1111/jnc.14218.

Schmidhuber, J. (2015). Deep learning in neural networks : An overview. *Neural Networks, 61*, 85–117. https://doi.org/10.1016/j.neunet.2014.09.003.

Simpraga, S., Alvarez-jimenez, R., Mansvelder, H. D., Van, J. M. A., Groeneveld, G. J., Poil, S., & Linkenkaer-hansen, K. (2017). EEG machine learning for accurate detection of cholinergic intervention and Alzheimer's disease. *Scientific Reports, 7*, 5775. https://doi.org/10.1038/s41598-017-06165-4.

Smith-Bindman, R., Miglioretti, D., Johnson, E., Lee, C., Feigelson, H., Flynn, M., … Williams, A. E. (2012). Use of diagnostic imaging studies and associated radiation exposure for patients enrolled in large integrated health care systems, 1996–2010. *JAMA, 307*(22), 2400–2409.

Strafella, C., Caputo, V., Galota, M. R., Zampatti, S., Marella, G., Mauriello, S., … Giardina, E. (2018). Application of precision medicine in neurodegenerative diseases. *Frontiers in Neurology, 9*(701). https://doi.org/10.3389/fneur.2018.00701.

Strimbu, K., & Tavel, J. A. (2010). What are biomarkers? *Current Opinion in HIV and AIDS, 5*(6), 463–466. https://doi.org/10.1097/COH.0b013e32833ed177.What.

Tuena, C., Serino, S., Dutriaux, L., Riva, G., & Piolino, P. (2019). Virtual enactment effect in young and aged populations: A systematic review. *Journal of Clinical Medicine, 8*, 620.

Valet, G. K., & Tárnok, A. (2003). Cytomics in predictive medicine. *Cytometry Part B: Clinical Cytometry, 53*(1), 1–3.

von Davier, A. A. (2017). Computational psychometrics in support of collaborative educational assessments. *Journal of Educational Measurement, 54*(1), 3–11.

Wang, E., Cho, W. C. S., Wong, C., & Liu, S. (2017). Disease biomarkers for precision medicine: Challenges and future opportunities. *Genomics, Proteomics & Bioinformatics, 15*(2), 57–58.

Wernick, M. N., Yang, Y., Brankov, J. G., Yourganov, G., & Stephen Strother, C. S. (2014). *Machine Learning in Medical Imaging, 27*(4), 25–38. https://doi.org/10.1109/MSP.2010.936730. Machine.

Chapter 6
Participatory Aspects of ICT Infrastructures for Cancer Management

Haridimos Kondylakis, Lefteris Koumakis, Ketti Mazzocco, Manolis Tsiknakis, and Kostas Marias

1 Introduction

As cancer research has come up with new, more effective treatments more and more cancer patients are being cured, and very many more enabled to live with their cancer. The disease is now frequently managed as a chronic illness requiring long-term surveillance and, in some cases, maintenance treatment. Cancer care occurs on a continuum that stretches from prevention to the end of life, with early detection, diagnosis, treatment, and survivorship in between. This implies a transformation in the nature of the existing healthcare model from reactive to preventive, and to personalized medicine. As a chronic illness, however, there is an urgent economic and pragmatic need for patients and families to manage their own care, and for the healthcare system to develop efficient strategies in supporting the achievement of this objective. Self-management support is defined as 'what health services do in order to aid and encourage people living with a long term condition to make daily decisions that improve health related behaviours and clinical and other outcomes'. Educating patients to self-management of disease strengthens health behaviours by promoting health literacy and collaborative decision-making skills, problem solving and action planning related to their condition. Such an approach is being embraced

---

H. Kondylakis (✉) · L. Koumakis · M. Tsiknakis · K. Marias
Computational BioMedicine Laboratory, Institute of Computer Science, Foundation for Research and Technology, Crete, Greece
e-mail: kondylak@ics.forth.gr; koumakis@ics.forth.gr; tsiknaki@ics.forth.gr; kmarias@ics.forth.gr

K. Mazzocco
Department of Oncology and Hemato-Oncology, University of Milan, Milan, Italy

Applied Research Division for Cognitive and Psychological Science, European Institute of Oncology (IEO) IRCCS, Milan, Italy
e-mail: ketti.mazzocco@ieo.it

G. Pravettoni, S. Triberti (eds.), *P5 eHealth: An Agenda for the Health Technologies of the Future*, https://doi.org/10.1007/978-3-030-27994-3_6

by government policies and in clinical practice, as demonstrated by the increasing number of initiatives and trials for patients' self-management.

Advances in information and communication technology (ICT), together with the recent spread of portable devices such as smartphones and tablets, offer the opportunity to re-design self-management. ICT can provide the means to transform the role of the patient from a passive recipient of healthcare services to an active, informed participant of medical decision-making processes in charge of his or her own well-being.

In this chapter, we review how this vision of building ICT platforms that promote and enhance the participation of all stakeholders involved in cancer management has been implemented in the context of five European research projects. Primarily they focus on the individual patient, empowering them and enabling better self-management, but also on the various care providers and health experts involved in the patient journey. Those projects focus on the transformation of the paternalistic model of patient–doctor to a new model that promotes the participatory aspects of all involved participants. We present achievements in the area of those five EU proposals, we identify the solutions provided and we discuss lessons learnt. Then we summarize and provide guidelines on the development of future ICT platforms.

The rest of this chapter is structured as follows: In Sect. 2, we elaborate on participatory aspects for cancer management and we highlight the need to transform the existing model, discussing also recent evidences on the area. Then in Sect. 3 we present experiences from five relevant EU projects (iManageCancer, MyHealthAvatar, p-Medicine, EURECA and INTEGRATE) and we elaborate on their approach to enable patients to participate in the management of their disease. Then in Sect. 4 we summarize the findings and we present directions for the development of future ICT platforms with a strong focus on further enhancing the patient participation on the management of their disease.

2 Participatory Aspects for Cancer Management

2.1 From Personalized to Participatory Medicine

Since the early 2000s, we are observing a profound revolution in the healthcare, with a shift in the medicine approach toward a predictive, preventive and personalized one, slowly moving towards the so-called 3P model (Hood et al. 2004; Weston and Hood 2004). Personalized medicine refers primarily to the genomic and molecular biology. Thanks to a unique combination of biological information, it is possible to design new pharmacological therapies tailored to the specific molecular picture of the patient.

Despite the important changes of this new approach, the underlying paradigm considered the patient still as a passive recipient of care, with the healthcare professionals as main actors. Three main aspects make this perspective suboptimal:

1) Medicine normally acts under uncertainty conditions, and some relevant information lies locked within the patient's body (Sox et al. 2013). To reduce uncertainty, besides the clinical examinations, some data can be obtained only from

the patient: doctors must rely on what the patient reports during the visits or using the patient reported outcomes measures (PROMs). In line with this perspective, the need to consider patients' knowledge, experiences and needs is not a mere ethical position, but it has also clinical consequences. As shown by Stacchiotti and Sommer, patients are not only passive care receivers but special collaborators that proactively can help clinicians and researchers reduce the aforementioned uncertainty (Stacchiotti and Sommer 2015) and find new therapeutic solutions.

2) The last 40 years has seen another initially slow but important shift in medicine: from a biomedical to a bio-psycho-social paradigm (Engel 1977; Inerney 2018). The World Health Organization has indeed defined health as a state of complete physical, mental, and social well-being, emphasizing the shift from the dominant paradigm with a focus on the disease to the new paradigm of wellness as a whole (WHO). The disease cannot be considered in isolation from its host: there is the need to understand and treat the disease considering the patient as a system, where the single parts strictly interact and produce an outcome that is something more than the sum of the single parts. In this perspective, personal psychological characteristics and social contexts interact with the biological factors in affecting the clinical outcomes. Consequently, the health professionals' aim within this paradigm is not anymore just to cure and increase life expectation, but to guarantee a good quality of life. Beside objective outcomes, the attention is paid also to subjective outcomes. The participation of the patient becomes therefore necessary, since the evaluation of what a life of quality means depends on the person's subjective values, priorities and preferences.
3) The spread of technology has made it easier for patients to access health information through the Internet. The constant growth of Internet as a source of health information (Morahan-Martin 2004; Internet World Stats 2016) (independently on the quality of the information) has contributed to make the patient a 'clinical expert', changing his/her role from passive recipient to active agent that wants to know and wants to participate in the decisions relevant for his/her health.

All these factors pushed for integrating the P3 medicine approach with other Ps, in particular a fourth P, standing for participatory (Hood and Friend 2011), and a fifth P that stands for psycho-cognitive (Gorini and Pravettoni 2011). In other words, the need for actively involving the patient in the care pathway has become a moral imperative (Pravettoni et al. 2016).

2.2 *Critical Factors of Participatory Medicine*

The Society for Participatory Medicine defined participatory medicine as 'a movement in which networked patients shift from being mere passengers to responsible drivers of their health, and in which providers encourage and value them as full partners' (Frydman 2010). Individual's genetic, molecular, cellular, organ and social networks will be combined into an overall 'network of networks', to give a detailed picture of the normal and disease-perturbed states. Following this approach, healthcare and wellness is not restricted anymore within the hospitals but moves into foundations and the patients' home. Chordoma Foundation (http://www.chordomafoundation.org) is a strong example of the power that the patient can have to make the difference in research for the cure of cancer or other fatal diseases, transforming, for example as in the case of Chordoma, a rare cancer to a not-so-rare cancer. Thanks to technology, indeed, Sommer, the executive director of Chordoma Foundation and personally diagnosed with Chordoma cancer, rounded up patients and researchers working on that specific cancer, optimizing the resources earlier scattered around the world, increasing awareness of the problem and breaking down barriers to progress.

Patients' participation in healthcare is relevant not only for improving research on new cancer treatments, but has positive effects on the patient's health condition. Barnato et al. (2007) noted that 'in an ideal world [...] patients would come to a cancer consultation armed with sufficient knowledge, clarity about their personal value, and the ability to engage in a thoughtful discussion about the pros and cons of treatment options. Providers, in turn, would be prepared to support their patients, armed with an understanding of the patient's knowledge gaps, personal values about possible outcomes and treatment preferences' (p. 627). The nature of malignant diseases such as cancer requires patients to learn about and comprehend the illness, make difficult decisions regarding ensuing treatment, and cope with the consequences of the illness. It has been found that having relevant information not only helps cancer patients to understand the disease, but it also facilitates their decision making and coping with the disease. Especially with cancer becoming a chronic disease, treatment places new demands on patients and families to manage their own care. A collaborative and interactive relationship between patients and health professionals can empower patients to take on responsibility for their condition with the appropriate clinical support. In this new concept of healthcare, clinician and patient are part of the same team: patients are empowered by more available information, and take a more active and responsible role, while clinicians welcome them as knowledgeable partners in clinical practice. The value of co-participation is particularly evident in the short- and long-term outcomes of shared decision making (Kane et al. 2014). Among the short-term outcomes are: satisfaction with and confidence in the made decision, satisfaction with physician–patient relationship, trust in the physician, increase in patient's self-efficacy and improvement in physical and emotional well-being. Long-term patient's outcomes are increases in treatment adherence, remission and quality of life. Despite the added value of the participation of patient in the information exchange and on decision-making process, its implementation in clinical practice is however still low. A systematic review (Kane et al. 2014) found that decision aids (DAs) improve patients' knowledge, reduce decisional conflict and motivate people to take a more active role in decision making. Informed decision making should combine the patients' personal values and the best available data. However, many patients have difficulties in associating these two components. Support tool such as a prompt list or decision aids can help them better manage the situation (Brown et al. 2013). However, DAs are usually standardized and are not necessarily adapted to the psycho-emotional state of the patient (Bekker et al. 2003; Davis et al. 2014).

2.3 *Psychological Factors as Moderators of Participatory Medicine*

In order to make the participatory approach efficient, we should open up space to explore patients' personal psychological, cognitive and social (familial) state (Gorini and Pravettoni 2011; Pravettoni and Gorini 2011). All these factors act as barriers or facilitators in patient's self-management.

Dealing with health information and decisions is not a straightforward process, especially if we consider that health literacy is generally poor among the population. Several studies have demonstrated that terminology is a barrier that decreases the level of engagement in the healthcare pathway (Keselman and Smith 2012) because of a poor understanding of medical documents, a high difficulty in adding non-understandable terms (their personal medical information) in Personal Health Records (PHR) (Genitsaridi et al. 2013, 2015), the discomfort in communicating with the physician about something they do not completely understand.

A first step in this direction is to understand how patients process information and what factors affect their capability to adapt and manage their illness and the decisions related to treatment, adherence, and lifestyles. The information selection and interpretation strongly depend on the patient's status quo, including knowledge, values, needs, believes and emotions, where emotions have a fundamental role in guiding the search for information and therefore the construction of preferences (Pravettoni et al. 2016b; Gorini et al. 2014).

In line with the aforementioned bio-psycho-social approach, besides a focus on the biological and psychological individual characteristics, it is important to consider social dynamics that can affect patient's self-management. The impact of a cancer diagnosis is indeed not limited to the individual; rather it influences their family and social network, which in turn can affect the patient's psychological state and therefore their empowerment. According to the family systems theory, a change in one member of the system affects the whole system (Von Bertalanffy 2003). In presence of an inadequate readjustment to the trauma, the system can develop clinically significant levels of distress, higher risk of developing psycho-social problems, high levels of conflict and low family cohesion (Van Schoors et al. 2015). The level and type of family adaptation eventually affects the patient's ability to cope with the illness.

The challenge of research in the last years, in line with the P5 approach, has been to build supportive environments that could be personalized for the specific patient. The multidisciplinary collaboration between oncologists, psychologists, engineers, IT professionals allowed the progress in the development of e-tools which can enhance patient empowerment and self-management, being also time-efficient and thus more easily integrated with the current clinical routine. What seemed an ideal in the traditional clinical practice becomes possible in the 'virtual' eHealth environment: to integrate all patient's data to provide a real personalized medical service. Coherently, information provided by physicians are tailored on the patient's psycho-cognitive profile; decision aids can support patient's choice according to his/her preferences and values, and that facilitate physician–patient shared decision making; specific smart applications support the patient to cope with cancer, manage their condition and adhere to healthy lifestyle; alerts from eHealth platforms inform physicians about clinical and psycho-emotional states of the patients.

3 ICT Solutions from Relevant EU Projects

3.1 iManageCancer

The iManageCancer project with the subtitle 'Empowering patients and strengthening self-management in cancer diseases', aims to provide a cancer disease self-management platform designed according to the specific needs of patient groups and focusing on the well-being of the cancer patient with special emphasis on psycho-emotional evaluation and self-motivated goals, as P5 approach shows. The platform is centred on a Personal Health Record that exploits recent advances on Health Avatars for the individual cancer patient surrounded by mHealth applications designed to encourage the patient, enhance clinician–patient communication, maximize compliance to therapy, inform about drug interactions, and contribute to the management of pain and other side effects of cancer treatment.

3.1.1 Technological Contribution

The iManageCancer platform was designed on clinical evidence and in close collaboration with clinical experts, IT specialists and patients and was assessed in clinical pilots with adult and paediatric cancer patients. The architecture of the technological contribution of the iManageCancer project is shown in Fig. 6.1.

Apart from the Personal Health Record that is the core component of the iManageCancer (Kondylakis et al. 2017a), the platform provides tools to assess adherence to therapy, physiological and psychological status and recommendations to the patient (Iatraki et al. 2018) according to his or her disease type and psycho-emotional status in order to promote a positive and healthier psycho-emotional state (Faccio et al. 2018) (Kazantzaki et al. 2016). The platform is further complemented by an expert system with formal self-management models oriented to decision support (Schera et al. 2018), serious games for children (Hoffmann and Wilson 2018) and adults (Zhang et al. 2018), e-Consent tool (Kondylakis et al. 2015c, 2017b) and anonymized data analysis (Koumakis et al. 2016b).

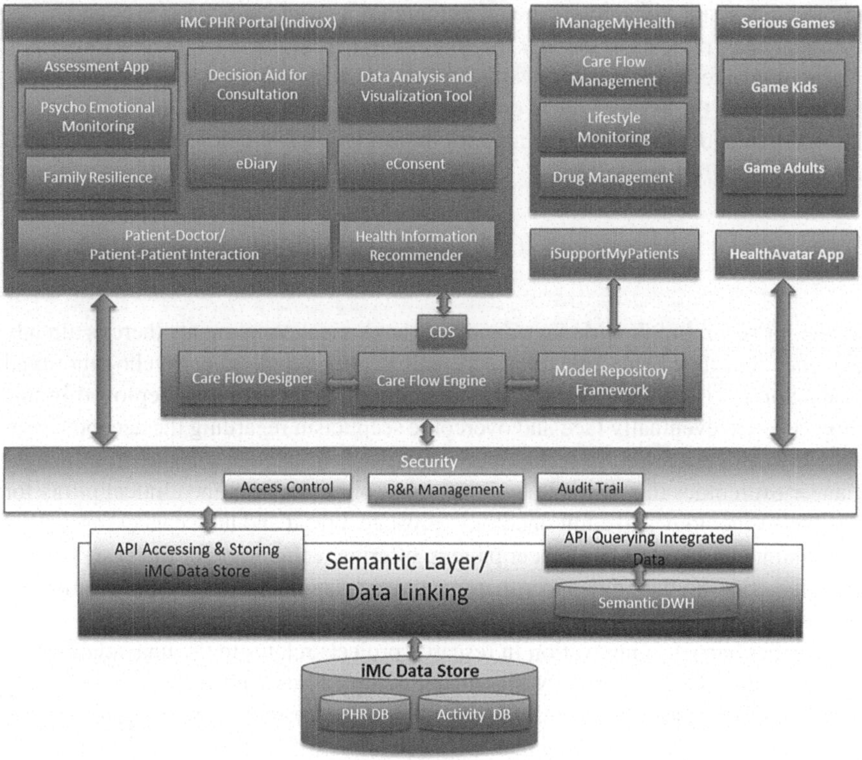

Fig. 6.1 The main components of the iManageCancer platform and their interactions

3.1.2 Participatory Aspect of the Developed Solution

iManageCancer aimed to arrange planned eHealth decision-making aids in cancer, promoting a self-aware and informed decision-making approach, compensating difficulties in shared decision-making approach with clinicians. In clinical practice, barriers in shared decision making are multiple. The most common ones are healthcare professionals' concerns about not having enough time, the perception that patient characteristics or the specific clinical situation were not conducive to shared decision making, the belief that some patients prefer a paternalistic approach without asking patients about their preferred role in decision making, and limited familiarity with shared decision making (Gravel et al. 2006).The proposed solution includes a novel approach for the collaborative management of cancer diseases with the informed and encouraged patient in a central role in the decision-making process.

Furthermore, the iManageCancer integrated mobile services act as the entry point for interactive disease self-management in close collaboration with the healthcare team. It advances disease management through reinforcement of the role of the patient in the management process, enabling better collaboration and interaction of informed patients with doctors, better planning of management processes and better compliance of patients to therapy through the mobile services of the platform.

Disruptive technologies for healthcare were also included such as serious games for monitoring the psychological dimensions of the disease. To this direction, games for children and adolescents but also for their relatives were developed and piloted for mobile platforms.

3.1.3 Lessons Learnt

While for several of the iManageCancer technological components there is already evidence that they can work for the benefit of the patient (e.g. psycho-emotional evaluation for improving therapy services etc.), the clinical pilots deployed in this project had to eventually face and overcome scepticism regarding the acceptance of such mHealth empowering technologies designed for the cancer patient. iManageCancer overcomes this obstacle by its serious commitment in the clinical pilots for paediatric oncology and adult oncology (prostate, breast and lung cancer) as well as the continuous focus on the cancer patient, offering technology for the best possible care, targeting on making cancer therapy a more personalized, continuous and participatory experience.

Another barrier to innovation in research projects relates to the unavailability of clinical data. There are usually significant complexities with respect to involving both clinicians and patients in real-life pilots. The large datasets available in the iManageCancer project and the real-life evaluations with patients and clinicians can eventually speed up innovation in areas such as data mining (Koumakis et al. 2018) and clinical decision support.

Results showed mixed evidences of improvements in patient empowerment due to lack of time and treatment-induced stress and psychological problems. Nevertheless, coping with cancer, mood and cancer resilience were improved for the trial arm using the platform. In addition, users recognized the usability and the usefulness of the developed platform. The different tools and services of the iManageCancer platform were developed and further optimized in several cycles implementing feedback of end-users and experiences from the pilots.

3.2 MyHealthAvatar

MyHealthAvatar project (http://www.myhealthavatar.eu/) (Kondylakis et al. 2015b; Maniadi et al. 2013) was an attempt to record digitally the health status of individual citizens. The goal was to create a digital representation of the user, a health avatar, acting as a mediator between the end-users and health-related data collections. It was designed as a lifetime companion for individual citizens that facilitates the collection, the access and the sustainability of health status information over the long term.

3.2.1 Technological Contribution

The architecture of the technological contribution of the MyHealthAvatar project is shown in Fig. 6.2. It consists of the following layers: (a) the data repository, (b) the semantic integration layer, (c) the auditing service, (d) the layer for linking with external sources, (e) the MyHealthAvatar toolbox and (f) the GUI (graphic user interface) layer. The data repository includes a data lake with various data sources that are available to the project, a tool/model repository and an imaging repository. Selected data out of this data lake are extracted, transformed and loaded onto a Virtuoso triple store where they are integrated. Data can also be extracted from

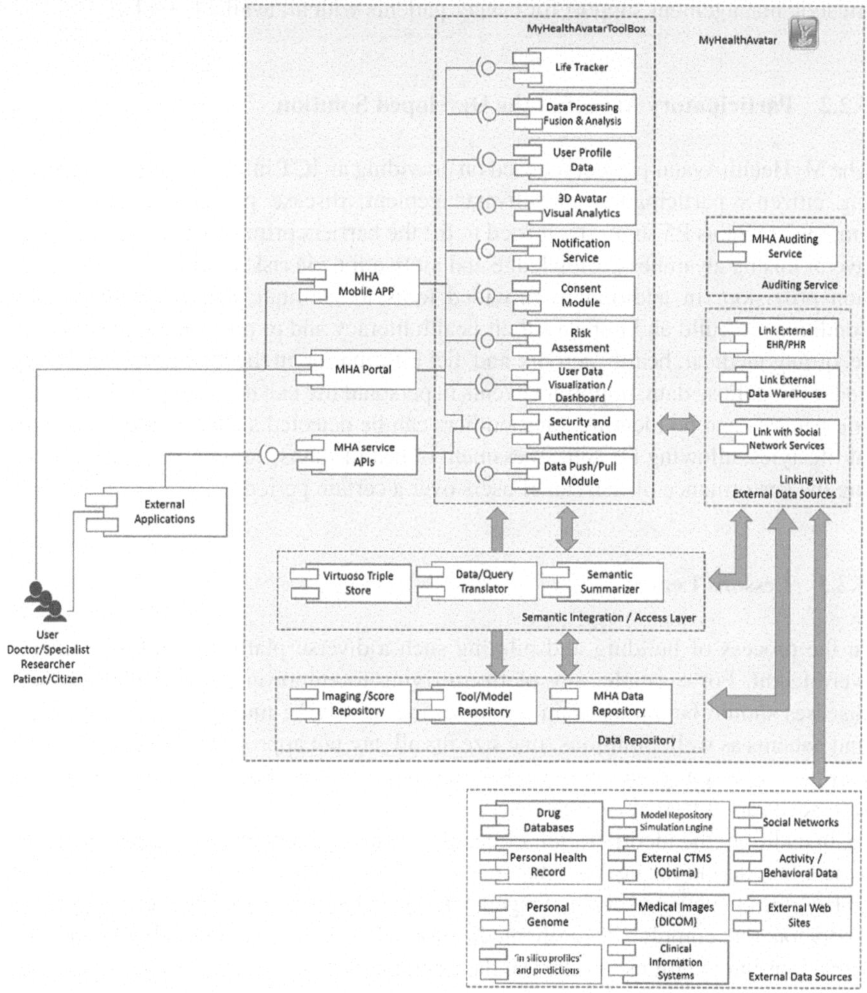

Fig. 6.2 The main components of the MyHealthAvatar platform and their interactions

external data sources using the various linking services. In addition to these data, the MyHealthAvatar toolbox includes all necessary services and implements the business logic to be presented through the GUI layer either using the MyHealthAvatar portal or the MyHealthAvatar Mobile app. The GUI layer facilitates and encourages self-monitoring and self-management via a number of different approaches (semi/automatic monitoring of individuals' steps count, calories consumption, active minutes, locations, movements, mood) through a 'virtual avatar', assists self-knowledge discovery through analysis and mining of personal health and activity data. Finally, it supports self-management of general health and well-being, and a range of chronic diseases via tailored intelligent tools (hypertension management, cardiovascular risk, diabetes, etc.). A specific branch of the platform (Zhang et al. 2018) is targeting lifestyle management support for cancer patients with all available tools.

3.2.2 Participatory Aspect of the Developed Solution

The MyHealthAvatar project focused on providing an ICT infrastructure for enhancing citizen's participation in self-management, disease prevention and patient empowerment as P5 suggests. It tried to lift the barriers primarily from the perspective of raising awareness, knowledge and motivation via risk appraisal and information provision. In addition, it provided tools to facilitate patients with chronic conditions to build and improve their health literacy and to provide a repository for recording medical, health, activity and diet information in the long term. Analyzing and mining those data, important events in personal life can be highlighted, personal life patterns can be identified and outliers can be detected such as sudden changes of lifestyles; allowing for self-assessment of health status; summarizing and reporting the performance of individual users over a certain period.

3.2.3 Lessons Learnt

In the process of building and piloting such a diverse platform, multiple lessons were learnt. For example, any platform trying to empower patients with chronic diseases should be validated in a real setting, involving multiple clinical partners and patients as well. Solutions 'one size fits all' are not appropriate in such a context and specific reconfiguration is needed for different types of diseases, as the information needs are different in each case.

In addition, the incorporation of health psychology models, is a key as they provide a foundation for health behaviour intervention. This enables the identification of key roles in patients' self-management, with a focus on their influence, and eventually on the compliance with medication plans, yielding individually tailored behaviour interventions to improve their compliance.

Finally, further investigation on usage of decision support tools is required. As gradually those tools mature, and their recommendations (Kondylakis et al. 2015a) are based on solid evidences, the confidence of the citizens will also increase enhancing their participation in their self-management.

3.3 *p-Medicine*

p-Medicine (From data sharing and integration via VPH models to personalized medicine) tried to formulate an open, modular framework of tools and services for efficient, secure sharing and handling of large personalized datasets (Marés et al. 2014). The platform enables demanding Virtual Physiological Human (VPH) multi-scale simulations (in silico oncology), builds standards-compliant tools and models for VPH research and provides tools for large-scale, privacy-preserving data and literature mining, a key component of VPH research. The project ensures that privacy, non-discrimination and access policies are aligned to maximize protection of and benefit to patients. The p-Medicine tools and technologies were validated within the concrete setting of advanced clinical research. Pilot cancer trials were conducted, based on clear research objectives, emphasizing the need to integrate multi-level datasets, in the domains of Wilms tumour, breast cancer and leukaemia. To sustain a self-supporting infrastructure, realistic use cases were built, demonstrating tangible results for clinicians.

3.3.1 Technological Contribution

Figure 6.3 shows the main components and their interdependency of the pmedicine system architecture from a clinical perspective.

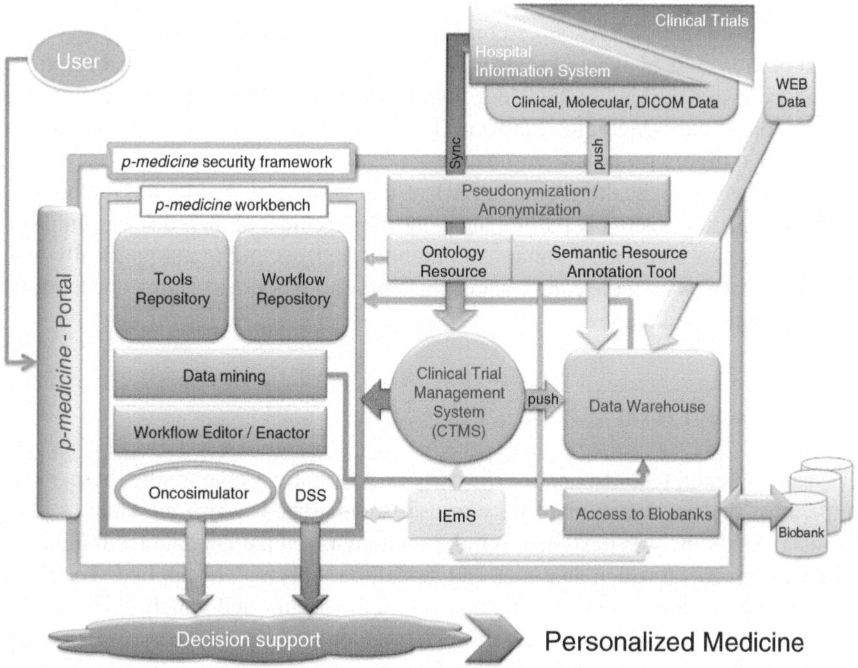

Fig. 6.3 The main components of the p-medicine platform and their interactions

A user is able to get access to p-medicine via a secure portal to use tools and workflows from the p-medicine workbench to execute his or her models by mining data from the data warehouse. The data warehouse is fed by data from Hospital Information Systems (HIS) or the integrated Clinical Trial Management Systems (CTMS) via a push service. The CTMS can synchronize with the HIS using a sync service. Data entering the p-medicine environment are pseudonymized/anonymized and semantically annotated (Sfakianaki et al. 2015). Access to external biobanks can be established and freely available data from the web can be stored in the data warehouse with the aid of literature mining (Potamias et al. 2005). Depending on the scenario, users are able to execute models (Sfakianakis et al. 2009), use the p-medicine Oncosimulator (Stamatakos et al. 2014), systems biology models (Koumakis et al. 2016a; Koumakis et al. 2017; Mehta et al. 2016) or they can use the Decision Support System (Bucur et al. 2016). In all cases results lead to personalized medicine via decision support. Patients as users of p-medicine can interact with the p-medicine environment via IEmS (Kondylakis et al. 2012), a collaborative environment for patient empowerment.

3.3.2 Participatory Aspect of the Developed Solution

The project aimed at providing clinical researchers with an infrastructure to support the requirements of modern clinical trials. From data collection and integration, to workflow design and result analysis, initial studies in the project detected some major points of interest for the area. There were specific needs to cover to alleviate end-users from the most resource-consuming tasks in their daily work. The combination of thorough analysis of scenarios, research on previously proposed solutions and an extensive tool and service development led, after four years of work, to the completion of the p-Medicine Platform. Intensive testing within real-world scenarios provided highly promising results.

A novel personal health record (PHR) system was developed within the project, enabling patients to actively participate in the management of their disease, employing psycho-emotional questionnaires to monitor patients and to automatically give recommendations to their carers about their psycho-emotional status and optimal communication guidelines.

3.3.3 Lessons Learnt

The patient health records, and the diversity of data sources comprising these, make imperative the development of easy-to-use, standardized health informatics platforms. p-Medicine was designed to link pseudonymized patient data from multiple clinical sources, on which analytics and modelling tools may be applied. The flexible, distributed nature of the system makes it highly robust and scalable. The implementation of an e-consent scenario through pseudonymization enables, unlike many similar platforms, results from the analytic processes that are found to have an impact on an individual patient, to be directly communicated, via the trusted third party, to the clinicians treating the patient.

Central to the challenges addressed by the p-medicine was the issue of semantic interoperability between production systems in both the clinical word (Electronic Health Record (EHR) systems) and the research domain (Clinical Trial Management Systems, Clinical Report Forms (CRF) systems, etc.). As a result, the issue of standards became a central activity in the project. Standards relate to both technical aspects of the systems developed as well as terminology and semantic aspects of this work. It was the intention of the project to integrate concepts from existing standards, models and architectures, while extending and refining them where appropriate and required. In achieving this objective the project had a dedicated task focusing on standards. The activities involved monitoring of standards development, critical review and assessment of their applicability in the p-medicine framework, refining such standards based on domain specific requirements.

3.4 EURECA

The goal of the EURECA project was to enable seamless, secure, scalable and consistent linkage of healthcare information residing in EHR systems with information in clinical research information systems, such as clinical trial systems, supporting the two currently separated worlds of clinical research and clinical practice to connect and benefit from each other. EURECA objective was to build an advanced, standards-based and scalable semantic integration environment, enabling seamless, secure and consistent bi-directional linking of clinical research and clinical care.

3.4.1 Technological Contribution

The aim of EURECA was to provide a framework of tools which can be easily interconnected in different configurations, tailored to the needs of different environments and end-users. To obtain this high flexibility, loose coupling and a service-orientated approach was chosen. The focus was thus on interoperability and interfacing in the architectural description. Modules and components designed and built within the project operated seamlessly through well-specified interfaces on different levels (i.e., interoperability on the level of IT-protocol, data format, information content, etc.). Figure 6.4 shows the architecture of the EURECA platform.

To obtain high flexibility, loose coupling and a service-orientated approach was chosen, emphasizing on interoperability and interfacing. Thus, EURECA architecture was determined by its interfaces. Modules and components designed and built within the project could operate together thanks to these well-specified interfaces at different levels. On the implementation level, EURECA internal services relied on SOAP as communication protocol.

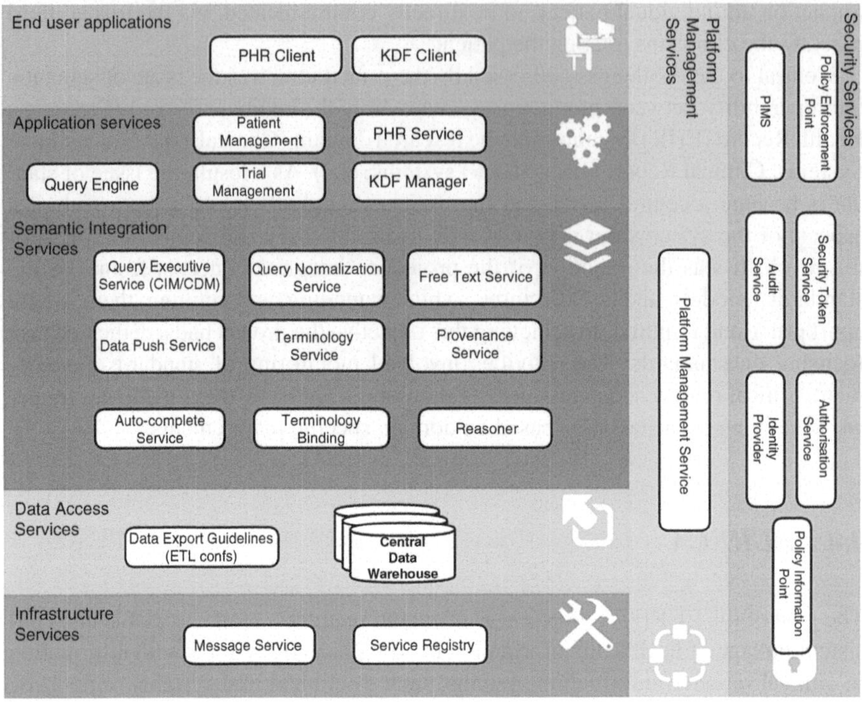

Fig. 6.4 The main components of the EURECA platform

The EURECA platform was designed as a multi-layered architecture, with responsibilities assigned to the various architectural layers. Every component designed within EURECA was mapped to one of these layers (or spanned over multiple layers). The architectural layers were:

- **End-User Applications**: The components situated in this layer could be seen as endpoints to the end-users of the system, presenting the underlying back-end functionality in an intuitive and user-friendly way. The components usually made use of a (advanced) graphical user interface (GUI) for displaying this (complex) back-end functionality.
- **Application Services**: This business layer provides the core functionality of the EURECA services as it houses a variety of application services. The components in this layer contained the functional algorithms that handled information exchange between the semantic integration layer and the presentation layer. Where possible, EURECA promoted the approach of providing re-usable services in the application layer.
- **Semantic Integration Services**: This layer utilized the ontology-based information model and translated or mapped the model to the underlying data and information sources. The semantic integration layer was abstracting the underlying data sources for the upper application layers.

- **Data Access Services**: This layer contained the various data and the metadata repositories. Services on this layer were responsible for the actual data access. The data warehouses exposed standardized query interfaces, and queries were expressed using the EURECA core dataset.
- **Infrastructure Services:** The components placed in this layer provided service communication and service management capabilities to other EURECA components.
- **Platform Management Services**: Included components that were enabling the management of the integration of the various components in the EURECA platform.
- **Security Services**: On an orthogonal axis, the security layer was connected to all other architectural layers. The EURECA security solution consisted of re-usable modular components that respectively dealt with authentication, authorization, audit and privacy enhancing (i.e. services oriented specifically at data privacy protection).

3.4.2 Participatory Aspects of the Developed Solution

EURECA supported more effective and efficient execution of clinical research by: (i) Allowing faster eligible patient identification and enrolment in clinical trials, (ii) providing access to the large amounts of patient data, (iii) enabling long-term follow-up of patients, (iv) avoiding the need for multiple data entry in the various clinical care. In order to achieve the aforementioned goals, EURECA platform provided the clinical research access—in a legally compliant and secure manner—to the large amounts of patient data collected in the EHR systems to be used for new hypotheses building and testing (e.g. to benefit rare diseases), cohort studies, as well as protocol feasibility.

At the core of the project was the semantic interoperability among EHR and clinical trial systems, consistent with existing standards, while managing the various sources of heterogeneity: technology, medical vocabulary, language, etc. This required the definition of sound information models describing the EHR and the clinical trial systems, and capturing the semantics of the clinical terms by standard terminology systems. The scalability of the solution was achieved by modularization, identifying core data subsets covering the chosen clinical domains. The project demonstrated and validated concepts developed in EURECA by implementing a set of software services and tools that were deployed in the context of pilot demonstrators. EURECA developed solutions that fulfill the data protection and security needs and the legal, ethical and regulatory requirements related to linking research and EHR data.

3.4.3 Lessons Learnt

The main barriers of secondary use of EHR data for research and of enabling a consistent feedback loop to care are the lack of common technology standards and concept terminologies. While solving the interoperability issue in healthcare at the generic level is not a realistic approach (Boyle and Levin 2008), EURECA aimed at semantic interoperability on domains of concepts (i.e. describing specific clinical areas). It began from disease- and treatment-related sets of concepts in the oncology domain and demonstrated the proposed solution in concrete clinical scenarios. On top of the achieved semantic interoperability software services and tools to support more efficient research, better care and improved patient safety were developed.

The approach taken in EURECA was to rely when possible on existing initiatives and previous efforts in terminology development and standardization. The viability of the solutions was demonstrated and developed by implementing a set of loosely coupled interconnected services/modules that have been deployed in the context of several pilot demonstrators in the cancer area, at healthcare sites.

The EURECA environment aims to provide several software services that help to securely interconnect the clinical trial systems and the electronic health record systems. This will bring several benefits, among which are early detection of patient safety issues and more efficient recruitment of eligible patients. Consistent linkage between CTS and EHRs will also help to significantly reduce the need for double data entry, which is currently often common practice.

3.5 *INTEGRATE*

The FP7 INTEGRATE project (http://www.fp7-integrate.eu/) focused on the development of innovative biomedical applications for streamlining the execution of clinical research on cancer (Kondylakis et al. 2016). This was achieved by enabling multi-disciplinary collaboration, contributing to the management and the large-scale sharing of multi-level heterogeneous datasets, and by developing new methodologies and predictive multi-scale models on cancer.

3.5.1 Technological Contribution

The technological infrastructure developed for the INTEGRATE project was composed of five layers as shown in Fig. 6.5.

On top, the presentation layer includes the various components that the end-users are using to access the patient screening application, the central pathology review, the cohort selection client and the analytical tools. The patient screening facilitates efficient identification of eligible patients for clinical trials through automatic matching of their characteristics and trial inclusion and exclusion criteria. Usually, patient data are described in free-text and this applies for trial exclusion and inclusion criteria. As such, automatic identification of eligible patients is a challenging task. On the other hand, enabling the collaboration and the participation of multiple clinical trial experts is an important challenge in modern multi-centric setting of clinical trials. The central pathology review tool enables high-quality, remote, decision making of multiple pathologists based on microscopy slides that are stored,

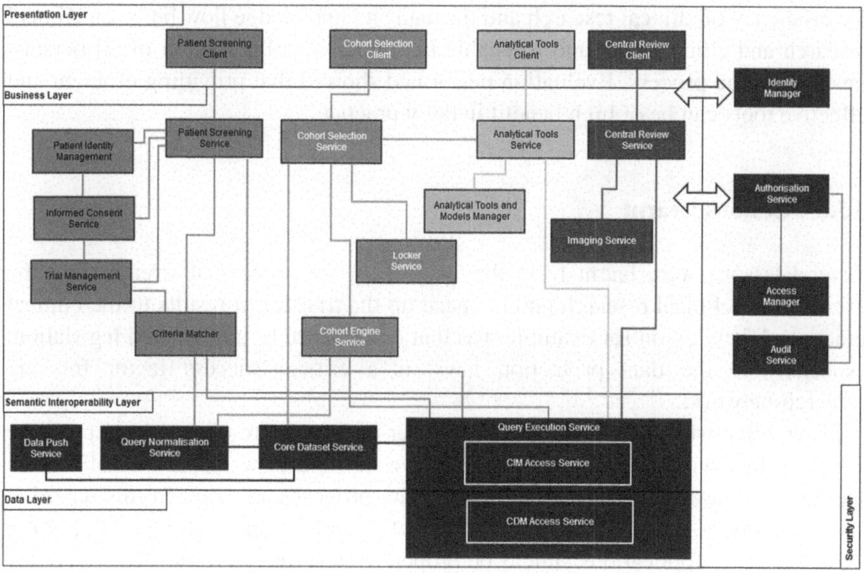

Fig. 6.5 A high-level view of the INTEGRATE technical Architecture (Kondylakis et al. 2016)

examined, annotated and commented online. Besides this, clinical researchers are able to formulate at run-time cohorts, based on multiple criteria available. In selected data can be visualized and analyzed in real time using the cohort selection and the analytical tools offered by the infrastructure.

Effective and efficient collaboration of clinical trial participants remains an important challenge in the modern multi-centric setting of such, post-genomic trials. The primary use of this Central Review for Pathology tool was to enhance the collaboration among groups of expert pathologists and to enable efficient, high-quality decision making for patients participating in a clinical trial.

The business layer includes all necessary services for patient screening, cohort selection, analytical services, imaging services and central review services. The semantic interoperability layer provides access to the homogenized data through an ontology. As such, the data layer includes the various data sources along with their corresponding metadata. Finally, a security layer establishes all necessary services for authentication, authorization and identity management.

3.5.2 Participatory Aspect of the Developed Solution

Although the specific project did not focus on enhancing the participatory aspect of the patient, it is interesting to see that it was focusing on the participatory aspect of multiple experts involved in multi-centric clinical research and trials in cancer (oncologists, research and trial nurses, researchers, bioinformaticians, pathologists, trial coordinators). More specifically, the project developed ICT solution to improve the efficiency of clinical research and the data and knowledge flow between clinical research and clinical care and to enable the effective collaboration of all persons involved in the process. Evaluation performed showed that providing efficient and effective tools can be of high benefit in daily practice.

3.5.3 Lessons Learnt

Several lessons were learnt from this project, in the process of streamlining the execution of clinical research and to speed up the transfer of results to the clinical practice. A key lesson for example was that compliance to trial-related legislation, especially to the data protection laws, is a critical success factor for any research-network.

Next, effective and efficient graphical user interfaces are of utmost importance when dealing with domain experts who have no time to waste and usually show inertia when new methods and approaches are proposed to them. In this regard, a really important lesson is that providing useful applications with nice GUI is not enough. Those applications should be properly integrated with the ICT tools they are already using and with their daily routine. In addition, service performance and stability are two keys in workflows with multiple participants with limited time.

4 Conclusions and Guidelines for Future Development

This chapter presented experiences from five European research projects, all focusing on enabling patients and related stakeholders to actively participate effectively and efficiently in the journey of the patient. We described the technological solutions that were built, we focused on the participatory aspect of each individual project and we described relevant lessons learnt.

As described, transforming the recent model of paternalistic care to a participatory one has many challenges, especially in a chronic illness domain like cancer, with multiple participants and stakeholders involved in a journey that might span multiple years. Although ICT and the proliferation of portable devices have the potential to lead to a leap forward, the steps needed come with many challenges. This is being reflected by the high number of research projects currently focusing on promoting specifically this participatory aspect. Capitalizing on the presented lessons learnt we can summarize the following guidelines:

User-centred design: Technological tools should always involve end-users in all phases of the development in an iterative process and that usability is equally important to the effectiveness of the tools in order to gain user acceptance. Patient should not only be employed to use the final product, but should actively co-design the developed solutions, as eventually they are the ones to use them.

Integration to daily workflow: In addition, in order to gain user acceptance the integration of the tools in the daily workflow of both the patients and the care providers is really important as they have limited time and they would like to minimize their potential involvements. Challenges related to semantic interoperability between production systems in both the clinical word (EHR systems) and the research domain (Clinical Trial Management Systems, CRF systems, etc.) should be resolved, whereas consistent linkage between clinical research and clinical practice will also help to significantly reduce the need for double data entry, which is currently often common practice. Specific attention should be paid to the fact that different professionals and organizations that participate in the patient's journey have different priorities (Schaller et al. 2016).

Mass scale: For long-term data collection of health-related data, individual participation at a mass scale is important. Such a comprehensive data collection will have a very strong clinical significance for diagnosis, prediction and individualized treatment, leading to significant evidence in health outcomes and quality of life.

Health psychology: Further involvement of the health psychology models will provide a foundation for health behaviour intervention, allowing the identification of key roles in patients' self-management, with a focus on their influence, and eventually on the compliance with medication plans, yielding individually tailored behaviour interventions.

Security and legal aspect: Securely interconnecting the clinical trial systems and the electronic health record systems can bring several benefits, among which are early detection of patient safety issues and more efficient recruitment of eligible patients. In addition, key challenges to be resolved are: assessing the validity of electronically given consent, data protection implications of access and use by third parties, the need for certification of apps/tools under the medical devices regime, and potential ex post facto liability in case of harm to users.

All these guidelines are essential, when creating ICT systems that are intended to be used by all involved participants in the journey of cancer management, but also for other chronic diseases as well, achieving eventually the P5 vision.

References

Barnato, A. E., Llewellyn-Thomas, H. A., Peters, E. M., Siminoff, L., Collins, E. D., & Barry, M. J. (2007). Communication and decision making in cancer care: Setting research priorities for decision support/patients' decision aids. *Medical Decision Making, 27*(5), 626–634.

Bekker, H. L., Hewison, J., & Thornton, J. G. (2003). Understanding why decision aidswork: Linking process with outcome. *Patient Education and Counseling, 50*(3), 323–329.

Boyle, P., & Levin, B. (2008). *World cancer report 2008*. IARC Press, International Agency for Research on Cancer.

Brown, R. F., et al. (2013). Perceptions of participation in a phase I, II, or III clinicaltrial among African American patients with cancer: what do refusers say? *Journal of Oncology Practice/ American Society of Clinical Oncology, 9*(6), 287–293.

Bucur, A., van Leeuwen, J., Christodoulou, N., Sigdel, K., Argyri, K., Koumakis, L., et al. (2016). Workflow-driven clinical decision support for personalized oncology. *BMC Medical Informatics and Decision Making, 16*(2), 87.

Davis, E. L., et al. (2014). An exploration of decision aid effectiveness: the im-pact ofpromoting affective vs: Deliberative processing on a health-related deci-sion. *Health Expectations, 18*, 2742–2752.

Engel, G. (1977). The need for a new medical model: A challenge for biomedical science. *Science, 196*, 126–129.

Faccio, F., Renzi, C., Crico, C., Kazantzaki, E., Kondylakis, H., Koumakis, L., et al. (2018). Development of an eHealth tool for cancer patients: monitoring psycho-emotional aspects with the Family Resilience (FaRe) Questionnaire. *ecancermedicalscience, 12*.

Frydman, G. (2010). A Patient-Centric Definition of Participatory Medicine. *e-patients.net*. Available online http://e-patients.net/archives/2010/04/a-patient-centric-definition-ofparticipatory-medicine.html, Accessed 20 Oct 2018.

Genitsaridi, I., Kondylakis, H., Koumakis, L., Marias, K., & Tsiknakis, M. (2013). Towards intelligent personal health record systems: Review, criteria and extensions. *Procedia Computer Science, 21*, 327–334.

Genitsaridi, I., Kondylakis, H., Koumakis, L., Marias, K., & Tsiknakis, M. (2015). Evaluation of personal health record systems through the lenses of EC research projects. *Computers in Biology and Medicine, 59*, 175–185.

Gorini, A., & Pravettoni, G. (2011). P5 medicine: a plus for a personalized approach to oncology. *Nature Review Clinical Oncology, 8*(7), 444.

Gorini, A., Mazzocco, K., Gandini, S., Munzone, E., McVie, G., & Pravettoni, G. (2014). Development and psychometric testing of a breast cancer patient profiling questionnaire. *Journal of Breast Cancer: Targets and Therapy, 2014*, 133–146.

Gravel, K., Légaré, F., & Graham, I. D. (2006). Barriers and facilitators to implementing shared decision-making in clinical practice: A systematic review of health professionals' perceptions. *Implementation Science*, 1–16.

Hoffmann, S., & Wilson, S. (2018). The role of serious games in the iManageCancer project. *ecancermedicalscience, 12*.

Hood, L., & Friend, S. H. (2011). Predictive, personalized, preventive, participative (P4) cancer medicine. *Nature Reviews. Clinical Oncology, 8*, 184–187.

Hood, L., Heath, J. R., Phelps, M. E., & Lin, B. (2004). Systems biology and new technologies enable predictive and preventative medicine. *Science, 306*, 640–643.

Iatraki, G., Kondylakis, H., Koumakis, L., Chatzimina, M., Kazantzaki, E., Marias, K., & Tsiknakis, M. (2018). Personal Health Information Recommender: implementing a tool for the empowerment of cancer patients. *ecancermedicalscience, 12*.

Inerney, S. J. M. (2018). Introducing the biopsychosocial model for good medicine and good doctors. *British Medical Journal, 324*, 1533.

Internet World Stats. (2016). World Internet Users and 2016 Population Stats, Internet World Users on June 30, 2016. *Miniwatts Marketing Group*. http://www.internetworldstats.com/stats.htm. Accessed 30 Oct 2018.

Kane, H. L., et al. (2014). Implementing and evaluating shared decision making in oncology practice. *CA: A Cancer Journal for Clinicians, 64*(6), 377–388.

Kazantzaki, E., Kondylakis, H., Koumakis, L., Marias, K., Tsiknakis, M., Fioretti, C., & Pravettoni, G. (2016). Psycho-emotional tools for better treatment adherence and therapeutic outcomes for cancer patients. *pHealth, 2016*, 129–134.

Keselman, A., & Smith, C. A. (2012). A classification of errors in lay comprehension of medical documents. *Journal of Biomedical Informatics, 45*, 1151–1163.

Kondylakis, H., Koumakis, L., Genitsaridi, E., Tsiknakis, M., Marias, K., Pravettoni, G., ... & Mazzocco, K. (2012, November). IEmS: A collaborative environment for patient empowerment. *Bioinformatics & Bioengineering (BIBE)*, 535–540. IEEE.

Kondylakis, H., Koumakis, L., Kazantzaki, E., Chatzimina, M., Psaraki, M., Marias, K., & Tsiknakis, M. (2015a). Patient empowerment through personal medical recommendations. In *MedInfo*, 1117.

Kondylakis, H., Spanakis, E. G., Sfakianakis, S., Sakkalis, V., Tsiknakis, M., Marias, K., Zhao, X., Yu, H.Q., Dong, F. (2015b). Digital patient: Personalized and translational data management through the MyHealthAvatar EU project. *EMBC*, 1397–1400.

Kondylakis, H., Flouris, G., Fundulaki, I., Papakonstantinou, V., & Tsiknakis, M. (2015c). Flexible access to patient data through e-Consent. In *Proceedings of the 5th EAI international conference on wireless mobile communication and healthcare* (pp. 263–266). ICST (Institute for Computer Sciences, Social-Informatics and Telecommunications Engineering).

Kondylakis, H., Claerhout, B., Mehta, K., Koumakis, L., van Leeuwen, J., Marias, K., Pérez-Rey, D., de Schepper, K., Tsiknakis, M., & Bucur, A. I. D. (2016). The INTEGRATE project: Delivering solutions for efficient multi-centric clinical research and trials. *Journal of Biomedical Informatics, 62*, 32–47.

Kondylakis, H., Koumakis, L., Hänold, S., Nwankwo, I., Forgó, N., Marias, K., et al. (2017b). Donor's support tool: Enabling informed secondary use of patient's biomaterial and personal data. *International Journal of Medical Informatics, 97*, 282–292.

Kondylakis, H., Bucur, A., Dong, F., Renzi, C., Manfrinati, A., Graf, N., & Tsiknakis, M. (2017a). iManagecancer: developing a platform for empowering patients and strengthening self-management in cancer diseases. *IEEE International Symposium on Computer-Based Medical Systems (CBMS), 2017*, 755–760.

Koumakis, L., Kanterakis, A., Kartsaki, E., Chatzimina, M., Zervakis, M., Tsiknakis, M., et al. (2016a). MinePath: Mining for phenotype differential sub-paths in molecular pathways. *PLoS Computational Biology, 12*(11), e1005187.

Koumakis, L., Kondylakis, H., Chatzimina, M., Iatraki, G., Argyropaidas, P., Kazantzaki, E., Tsiknakis, M., Kiefer, S., Marias, K. (2016b). Designing smart analytical data services for a personal health framework. *pHealth*, 123–128.

Koumakis, L., Roussos, P., & Potamias, G. (2017). minepath. org: A free interactive pathway analysis web server. *Nucleic Acids Research, 45*(W1), W116–W121.

Koumakis, L., Kondylakis, H., Katehakis, D. G., Iatraki, G., Argyropaidas, P., Hatzimina, M., & Marias, K. (2018). A content-aware analytics framework for open health data. In *Precision Medicine Powered by pHealth and Connected Health,* 59–64.

Maniadi, E., Kondylakis, H., Spanakis, E., Spanakis, M., Tsiknakis, M., Marias, K., Dong, F. (2013). Designing a digital patient avatar in the context of the MyHealthAvatar project initiative. *BIBE*, 1–4.

Marés, J., Shamardin, L., Weiler, G., Anguita, A., Sfakianakis, S., Neri, E., ... & Coveney, P. V. (2014). p-medicine: A medical informatics platform for integrated large scale heterogeneous patient data. In *AMIA Annual Symposium Proceedings*, 2014, 872.

Mehta, S., Hughes, N. P., Li, S., Jubb, A., Adams, R., Lord, S., et al. (2016). Radiogenomics monitoring in breast cancer identifies metabolism and immune checkpoints as early actionable mechanisms of resistance to anti-angiogenic treatment. *eBioMedicine, 10*, 109–116.

Morahan-Martin, J.M. (2004). How internet users find, evaluate, and use online health information: A cross-cultural review. *Cyberpsychol Behav.*, 7, 497–10.

Potamias, G., Koumakis, L., & Moustakis, V. (2005). Mining XML clinical data: The HealthObs system. *Ingénierie des systèmes d'information, 10*(1), 59–79.

Pravettoni, G., & Gorini, A. (2011). A P5 cancer medicine approach: Why personalized medicine cannot ignore psychology. *Journal of Evaluation in Clinical Practice, 17*, 594–596.

Pravettoni, G., Cutica, I., Righetti, S., & Mazzocco, K. (2016). Decisions and the involvement of cancer patient survivors: a moral imperative. *Journal of Healthcare Leadership, 8*, 121.

Pravettoni, G., Mazzocco, K., Gorini, A., & Curigliano, G. (2016b). Understanding cognitive processes behind acceptance or refusal of phase I trials. *Critical Re-views in Oncology/Hematology, 100*, 69–73.

Schaller, S., Marinova-Schmidt, V., Setzer, M., Kondylakis, H., Griebel, L., Sedlmayr, M., et al. (2016). Usefulness of a tailored eHealth service for informal caregivers and professionals in the dementia treatment and care setting: the eHealthMonitor Dementia Portal. *JMIR Research Protocols, 5*(2).

Schera, F., Schäfer, M., Bucur, A., van Leeuwen, J., Ngantchjon, E. H., Graf, N., Kondylakis, H., Koumakis, L., Marias, K., & Kiefer, S. (2018). iManageMyHealth and iSupportMyPatients: Mobile decision support and health management apps for cancer patients and their doctors. *ecancermedicalscience, 12*.

Sfakianaki, P., Koumakis, L., Sfakianakis, S., Iatraki, G., Zacharioudakis, G., Graf, N., Marias, K., & Tsiknakis, M. (2015). Semantic biomedical resource discovery: A Natural Language Processing framework. *BMC Medical Informatics and Decision Making, 15*(1), 77.

Sfakianakis, S., Koumakis, L., Zacharioudakis, G., Tsiknakis, M. (2009). Web-based authoring and secure enactment of bioinformatics workflows. In *Grid and Pervasive Computing Conference*, 88–95.

Sox, H. C., Higgins, M. C., Owens, D. K. (2013). *Medical decision making*.

Stacchiotti, S., & Sommer, J. (2015). Building a global consensus approach to chordoma: A position paper from the medical and patient community. *The Lancet Oncology, 16*(2), e71–e83.

Stamatakos, G., Dionysiou, D., Lunzer, A., Belleman, R., Kolokotroni, E., Georgiadi, E., et al. (2014). The technologically integrated oncosimulator: Combining multiscale cancer modeling with information technology in the in silico oncology context. *IEEE Journal of Biomedical and Health Informatics, 18*(3), 840–854.

Van Schoors, M., Caes, L., Verhofstadt, L. L., Goubert, L., & Alderfer, M. A. (2015). Systematic review: Family resilience after pediatric cancer diagnosis. *Journal of Pediatric Psychology, 40*(9), 856–868.

Von Bertalanffy, L. (2003). General system theory. In *The science of synthesis: Exploring the social implications of general systems theory* (p. 304). Boulder: University Press of Colorado.

Weston, A. D., & Hood, L. (2004). Systems biology, proteomics, and the future of health care: Toward predictive, preventative, and personalized medicine. *Journal of Proteome Research, 3*, 179–196.

World Health Organization. [webpage on the Internet]. WHO definition of health. Available at https://www.who.int/about/mission/en/. Accessed October 20, 2018.

Zhang, X., Deng, Z., Parvinzamir, F., & Dong, F. (2018). MyHealthAvatar lifestyle management support for cancer patients. *ecancermedicalscience*, 12.

Chapter 7
Psycho-cognitive Factors Orienting eHealth Development and Evaluation

Alessandra Gorini, Enrico Gianluca Caiani, and Gabriella Pravettoni

1 The P5 and the Personomics Approach

"Individuality of human beings affects predisposition to disease and response to treatment" (Potter, 1988; Sykiotis, Kalliolias, & Papavassiliou, 2005), stated Hippocrates in the fifth century BC, becoming the first known physician mentioning the relevance of a personalized approach to diagnosis and treatment. Many centuries later, personalized medicine has gained increasing attention (Britten, Pope, Halford, & Richeldi, 2016; Brownell et al., 2016), applying the Hippocratian vision to the need of "delivering the right treatment to the right patient at the right time" (MRC, 2017) (cf. Chap. 4).

Starting from the individuality of human beings—and to further enrich the personalized medicine approach—that is mainly based on the biological characterization of each individual, some years ago we proposed the P5 approach (Gorini & Pravettoni, 2011; Pravettoni & Gorini, 2011). The fifth P (that followed the other four P's: *p*redictive, *p*ersonalized, *p*reventive, and *p*articipatory (Hood & Friend, 2011)) indicated the *p*sycho-cognitive aspects that characterize a patient not only as a biological and genetic entity, but also as a person with specific needs and values, habits and behaviors, hopes and fears, beliefs, personality, and cognitive dispositions. Introducing the fifth P, we underlined the need of integrating all these aspects with biological and genetic information in order to empower the patient, increase

A. Gorini (✉) · G. Pravettoni
Department of Oncology and Hemato-Oncology, University of Milan, Milan, Italy

Applied Research Division for Cognitive and Psychological Science,
European Institute of Oncology (IEO) IRCCS, Milan, Italy
e-mail: alessandra.gorini@unimi.it; gabriella.pravettoni@ieo.it

E. G. Caiani
Department of Electronics, Information and Bioengineering, Politecnico di Milano,
Milano, Italy
e-mail: enrico.caiani@polimi.it

G. Pravettoni, S. Triberti (eds.), *P5 eHealth: An Agenda for the Health Technologies of the Future*, https://doi.org/10.1007/978-3-030-27994-3_7

his/her quality of life (QOL) and transform him/her from a passive recipient of care into an active decision-maker during the entire treatment process (Joseph-Williams, Elwyn & Edwards, 2014) (cfr. Chap. 1).

In line with this patient-centered approach, a few years later, the term "personomics" was introduced (Ziegelstein, 2015). Inspired by the other "-omics," including genomics, proteomics, metabolomics, epigenomics, and pharmacogenomics, created to characterize patients by their biological uniqueness and to provide more precisely tailored diagnostics and therapeutics, personomics refers to the patient's unique psychosocial situation and life circumstances that may alter disease behavior and response to treatment (Ziegelstein, 2015). In accordance with the previous P5 approach, personomics distinguishes individuals not only by their biological variability, but also by their psychological characteristics, health beliefs, social support networks, education, socioeconomic status, health literacy, and all the other life conditions and events that may have important consequences on when and how a certain health condition will manifest in that individual and how it will respond to treatment (Ziegelstein, 2015). As the other -omics, these individual characteristics are critical to patient care, being useful for a better understanding of the pathogenesis and treatment of disease and allowing a more personalized care that takes into account the patient's internal world and external life circumstances.

By embracing the P5 and the personomics approaches, non-pharmacological interventions, including, among others, psychological support, a greater involvement of patients in shared decision making, and lifestyle coaching, appear to be relevant to reinforce the effects induced by traditional pharmacological treatments. Assessing the individual needs and perspectives, together with the patient's psychological attitudes and preferences may be also relevant to improve his/her treatment adherence, satisfaction, and, overall, his or her short- and long-term quality of life. Moreover, since such personal characteristics can change over time, or because of the presence of an illness or, again, its progression or recovery, an iterative evaluation of the individual patient may become a key feature for an effective personalized disease management (cfr. Chap. 3).

In traditional care paradigms, patients are physically evaluated when the diagnosis is established, and, only when necessary, at one or more follow-ups. Sometimes, psychological and/or quality of life evaluations are also performed depending on the patient's illness and local guidelines. Nevertheless, such evaluations, when present, are not sufficient to guarantee the right attention to the above individual factors and do not allow a long-term monitoring of the patient's characteristics and evolution. Moreover, time and cost constraints, other than patients' limitations and difficulties, prevent the application of the P5 approach in the actual clinical practice.

According to the P5 and the personomics approaches, collecting organized patient's input throughout the entire disease course is important for different reasons:

- To correlate psychological variables and quality of life with physical events, clinical state, and clinical recurrences

- To better respect the patient's needs and preferences to not lose treatment adherence
- To provide better tailored treatments
- To maintain a contact with patients during and after recovery
- To empower patients in improving their understanding of their health conditions and in making them actively involved in the management of their own disease

2 The Key Elements for the P5-Personomics Approach

What are the key elements of the P5-personomics approach and how can they be collected? Which instruments can be used by physicians to understand the patient as an individual?

The National Institute for Health and Clinical Excellence (NICE) has proposed a guideline document ((UK), 2012) that outlines 5 areas containing the elements of knowing the (adult) patient as an individual (p. 48). These areas include the consideration of:

1. How clinical conditions affect the person and how the person's situations and experiences affect his/her condition and treatment.
2. How the patient's life circumstances affect his/her treatment involvement and experiences, and his/her lifestyle choices.
3. How the patient's concerns, values, and preferences affect the way he/she engages with the treatment experience.
4. How the patient's psychological, social, spiritual needs affect his/her condition and treatment.
5. They also include an admonition to clinicians not to make assumptions about the patient based on appearance.

To answer the second question as to how such information can be collected, the most intuitive solution would be to interview each patient for as much time as possible. Unfortunately, this is not a feasible solution in the everyday clinical practice for the following reasons:

- Physicians have not enough time to investigate such aspects.
- Collecting this information requires different methods compared to those used to investigate medical symptoms.
- One single interview is not sufficient to implement a new model of cure based on the P5 approach.

3 Solutions Come from the eHealth Apps

A very promising approach to solve the above limitations and to collect as much data as possible involving patients in managing their health comes from eHealth. eHealth solutions have been considered in the last two decades as the "holy grail," able (if properly implemented and scaled up) to reduce healthcare costs (cfr. Chap. 1), and improve patient experience while maintaining adequate levels of care (Tang and Lansky 2005; Bradford & Palmer 2016) (cfr. Chap. 4). In particular, eHealth solutions provide the basis for "participatory health" (cfr. Chap. 6), in which active involvement of all the involved parties—the patient, caregivers, and healthcare professionals alike—is encouraged. This assumes particular importance in the context of searching for innovative ways of supporting chronic patients, where it is fundamental to keep under control the underlying pathology and detect as early as possible the signs of worsening in order to anticipate countermeasures and prevent possible hospitalization. Thanks to the developments in the field of information and communication technology (ICT) observed in the last years, in particular with the large penetration of mobile cellular phone technology in the global market and its ubiquitous access to the World Wide Web, a large proportion of the world population has now access to and uses the Internet in their daily lives (via, e.g., a PC, tablet, wearables, and/or smartphone), thus finally providing the tools for the "holy grail" to exploit its potentials within healthcare (Internet World Stats, 2018; Kay et al., 2011).

This technologically permeated background, if properly utilized in the context of clinical medicine, has the potential to switch the way healthcare is provided from a paternalistic model to a collaborative approach, by means of self-management, shared decision making, and a coaching relation between the physician and the patient (Mead and Bower, 2000; Bacigalupe & Askari, 2013) (cfr. Chap. 4). In this way, the focus of healthcare could be moved from management of acute episodes to secondary prevention, and also to primary prevention (cfr. Chap. 3), physical fitness, nutrition, mental health, end-of-life care, home-care, and other fields related to an individual's health.

4 Digital Health in the Patient's Journey

Indeed, the use of technology for health is already permeating the patient journey, from prevention to treatment: while there are no diseases, access to specific tools such as mobile applications (or "apps") could increase knowledge about possible risks associated to incorrect lifestyle behaviors and help in increasing levels of wellness through self-monitoring of exercise and fitness, diet and nutrition, alcohol moderation, and smoking cessation.

Once symptoms of a disease are manifested, a plethora of patient experience tools are available: searching related keywords on the web, specific apps for symptom checking, social media to share concerns, and tools to find specialized centers if necessary.

In the process of clinical decision making, the physician could base the diagnosis on data acquired directly by the patient using smartphone embedded sensors or connected medical devices that have the potential to record possible pathologic phenomena when they manifested, if symptomatic (e.g., for atrial fibrillation (Halcox et al., 2017), thus overcoming some existing limitations of well-established diagnostic Holter ECG technology).

Once the diagnosis has been established, the physician may recommend digital tools for condition monitoring, such as app-supported disease management programs, connected sensors for remote monitoring and rehabilitation programs, or apps for psychological and cognitive profiling, and for any use case across the patient journey. In addition, patients could share their experiences, success and failure stories in patient's forum groups specific for the underlying pathology. In the context of treatment, medication management and adherence could be improved by utilizing digital tools, from simple reminders activated through the smartphone to more advanced electronic medication packaging (EMP), or solutions based on active patient involvement and artificial intelligence.

4.1 A Possible Scenario

Taking into account the P5 approach, such tools could be perhaps structured on the basis of the NICE guidelines, to be used by the patient both during the acute and the chronic phase of the illness. Organized in different areas, they can be used to:

1. Fill health journal, allowing users to record their clinical parameters directly or from remote monitoring tools.
2. Write diaries of life events that can have a significant impact on the individual well-being and quality of life. They include negative or stressful events occurring in everyday working or personal life, health-related events, illness recurrences, and any kind of event that is perceived as negative by the individual.
3. Collect the patient's concerns about the treatment experience, such as treatment side effects, or patient's complaints including physical or behavioral aspects induced by treatments.
4. Regularly collect information about the patient's social conditions and psychological status. Individual characteristics, such as personality traits, decision-making style, emotional profile, as well psychological dimensions, such as the presence of stress, anxiety, depression, etc, and the presence of protective or negative social conditions (social support or social isolation, etc.) are collected in this area.

All this information may be collected through monitoring tools and periodic remote administrations of specific questionnaires starting from the acute phase of the illness (if possible) for as long a time as possible in order to provide long-term monitoring of the patient, from the acute to the chronic phase.

Specific algorithms are then needed to put together information obtained from the different areas in order to integrate physical, environmental, and psychological factors into explanatory and possibly predictive models.

At the same time, periodic reports for patients and physicians may be created by the system in order to make the patient aware of his/her condition and to alert the physicians when unexpected or worrying events or health changes occur.

A comprehensive monitoring program, consisting of an eHealth app collecting different patient information may have the potential to improve trial design, enhance self-management, allow for early treatment adaption to minimize side effects, reduce hospital admissions, and, in general, improve personalized management and long-term QOL. Only by integrating biological information with patient-reported and patient-collected information, will we be able to realize truly personalized treatment, preventing clinicians from making assumptions about the patient based on appearance, as suggested by the fifth point of the NICE guidelines.

5 The Importance of Patient Education

Due to the availability of medical information through an incredible number of sources, a deep cultural change has been manifested, and described by the term of apomediation (Eysenbach, 2008) that is the process of disintermediation, where previous intermediaries (e.g., healthcare professionals) are functionally bypassed by new apomediaries (i.e., the web, online groups, GoogleSearch, etc.) in guiding the citizens' access to health information.

To appreciate the relevance of this phenomenon, this open access to information through technology could be compared to what happened after the introduction of movable-type printing press by Gutenberg in 1439, which led later to the era of mass communication in Renaissance Europe. This invention, by increasing literacy, permanently altered the structure of the society by the relatively unrestricted circulation of information and revolutionary ideas, thus threatening the power of political and religious authorities and breaking the education and learning monopoly of the literate elite, thereby bolstering the emerging middle class.

In the medical information context, while increasing patient literacy is a positive factor, the chief ethical concern regarding apomediation is that incorrect ideas or potentially dangerous practices will take hold. As observed previously, patient education is a lifelong program, where technology can enhance the learning process, but reliable content is the key. Examples of possible consequences related to these cultural changes are represented by the information overload while searching information through Internet (e.g., 770 million results are returned by Google when searching for "cancer" and 389 million when searching for "diabetes"), or by the incredible proliferation of apps in the "Medical" and "Health & Fitness" categories in the app stores: the patient is potentially left alone in the process of choosing which information to rely on, or which app to adopt that best suits her/his needs, with the risk of trusting unreliable sources or using apps with claims not supported by validation for accuracy and efficacy.

In the process of patient empowerment, defined as the acquisition of motivation and ability that patients might use to be involved or participate in decision making (Fumagalli et al., 2015), patient education becomes a critical goal for patient enablement, that is, the acquisition of knowledge and skills for meaningful self-management.

Patient education aims to increase the level of health literacy, defined as the ability of the patient to obtain, read, understand, and use healthcare information to make appropriate health decisions and follow instructions for treatment and self-care (Sørensen, et al., 2012; Mårtensson and Hensing, 2012). Indeed, patient literacy constitutes the first step to properly understand health concepts, and it has been indicated by the World Health Organization as one of the social and economic factors impacting on adherence, defined as the extent to which the persons' behavior corresponds with agreed recommendations from a healthcare provider (Adherence to long-term therapies. Evidence for action, WHO 2003). To effectively utilize mHealth technology, health literacy is not enough, as digital literacy, that is, the ability to locate, organize, understand, evaluate, and analyze information using digital technology, needs to be ensured. These two abilities have been lately summarized in the concept of digital health (eHealth) literacy as the ability to seek, find, understand, and appraise health information from electronic sources and apply the knowledge gained to addressing or solving a health problem (Norman and Skinner, 2006). As a recent EU-funded project (Health Literacy Europe) has highlighted, health literacy cannot be taken for granted as, of the eight countries (Austria, Bulgaria, Germany, Greece, Ireland, the Netherlands, Poland, Spain) surveyed, only the Netherlands showed less than 40% of the studied population with inadequate or problematic levels, while the other countries had higher values, with extremes found in Spain (58.5%) and Bulgaria (62.1%).

Considering that the main cause of medical errors have been attributed to communication-related origins (Hughes and Ortiz, 2005), the ability of the patient to fully understand medical recommendations given by the physician during the consultation appears crucial: in Kessels (2003) it was reported that from the given medical information, 40–80% is immediately forgotten, while half retained is incorrect. To improve physician–patient communication, the teach-back assessment has been proposed as a method to confirm patient's understanding of medication and treatment recommendations (Porter et al., 2016). In this context, digital technologies provide new opportunities also for physicians to get used to this approach, with online learning modules freely available through the Internet (Abrams et al., 2012) or for the patient, with video recorded outpatient clinic sessions accessible for the patient via patient portal, as recently implemented at the Erasmus Medical Center in Rotterdam.

In order to define the baseline level for comparison after exposure to the educational interventions to determine its effectiveness, it is important to assess patient health literacy. In literature, different assessment tools have been proposed; for example, the Rapid Estimate of Adult Literacy in Medicine (REALM) (Davis et al.,

1993), or the Test of Functional Health Literacy in Adults (TOHFLA) (Parker et al., 1995), designed to measure both reading comprehension and numeracy to assess adult literacy in the healthcare setting. In the context of eHealth and health informatics for patients or for the public, it is crucial to be aware of who the final user really is and what characteristics he/she has that might impact on eHealth design and implementation: digital health (eHealth) literacy needs to be assessed. The foundations of the eHealth literacy concept are based in part on social cognitive and self-efficacy theories, which promote competencies and confidence as precursors to behavior change and skill development. eHealth literacy includes six core skills, or literacies: (1) traditional literacy; (2) health literacy; (3) information literacy; (4) scientific literacy; (5) media literacy; (6) computer literacy. The eHealth Literacy Scale (eHEALS) is a self-report tool composed of eight questions that can be administered by a health professional and is based on an individual's perception of his/her own skills and knowledge within each measured domain (Norman and Skinner, 2006).

6 Persuasive Design Technology

Research has proven that by means of technology, it is possible to help people to change their thoughts, improve their behavior and gain better health and well-being. Cognitive behavior psychology aims to explain, predict, and change our behavior using processes that are going on in the mind. In 1958, Albert Ellis developed one of the first cognitive behavior theories explaining how and what kind of cognitions (i.e., beliefs and thoughts) can change behavior. Since then, several theories for behavior change have been developed, thus prescribing what factors must be first influenced.

Behavior change is about persuasion, therefore behavior change techniques are often persuasive strategies as well. In the last decades, technology is used more and more as a vehicle for persuasion, because of its interactivity and adaptability. Compared to human persuasion, technology solutions present several advantages:

- Persistence: technology does not get tired of trying to persuade someone, and it can continue indefinitely.
- Anonymity: when talking to a human persuader, it is impossible to stay anonymous, while with technology this is easier, thus representing a huge advantage for sensitive subjects (i.e., psychological problems or substance abuse).
- Ability to manage large volumes of data: technology's ability to process huge volumes of data in a short time gives more persuasive power, as technology can back up a certain message with the data that supports it.
- Scalability: people can only reach a limited number of other people; using technology, many more people can be reached without a large increase in cost.

- Ubiquity: technology can be everywhere, even in places where a human persuader cannot be allowed to be. As for many behavior change techniques, effective timing of message delivering is crucial, so ubiquity represents a pivotal characteristic to modify existing behaviours;
- Multimodality: technology can present information in many different ways, including text, audio, and video, thus matching each person's individual preferences to the persuasive methods it uses.

In the late 1990s, the use of technology to persuade the users to change their behavior was first defined by Fogg (2002), and more recently persuasive systems were defined as "computerized software or information systems designed to reinforce, change or shape attitudes or behaviours or both without using coercion or deception" (Oinas-Kukkonen and Harjumaa 2018).

Technology can act in persuading throughout several different techniques:

- Informing: individuals have to learn the presented information, in order for this information to be remembered.
- Reinforcement: desired behaviour should be rewarded/reinforced as quickly as possible upon its performance.
- Discussing: individuals share their thinking processes and beliefs among each other.
- Social comparison: individuals are stimulated to compare themselves with individuals from other groups that perform the desirable behavior.
- Fear appeal: materials (i.e., images or texts that elicit fear) are presented and should appeal fear to individuals of the target group; typically, fear appeals are effective to a certain extent only, because, when reaching a high level of elicited fear, target users could avoid the issue instead of considering it.
- Skills training: individuals learn from practicing behavior by themselves, and practice improves their confidence.

In the context of the P5 approach, by using the persuasive power of technology, eHealth solutions can be made more effective, as people are more adherent to eHealth interventions when more persuasive elements are used (Kelders & Van Gemert-Pijnen, 2013). The Persuasive System Design (PSD) model (Oinas-Kukkonen and Harjumaa 2018) represents a state-of-the-art approach for designing and evaluating persuasive systems. It is applicable to systems that are designed to form, alter, or reinforce attitudes, behaviors, or an act of compliance without using deception, coercion, or inducements, that is, it is well suited for the design of eHealth technologies.

The PSD model assumes several principles common to all persuasive systems, as regards the ways that people can be persuaded by means of technology:

- Technology is never neutral, but has always an intention.
- People like their views and behavior to be organized and consistent: if systems support the making of commitments, then users are more likely to be persuaded to follow these commitments.

- Persuasion is often incremental: behavior change never takes place at once, but in small steps.
- Direct and indirect routes: paying attention (consciously or unconsciously) is very important when changing behavior.

As regards the characteristics that a technology should have in order to effectively persuade people, these can be listed as:

- Unobtrusive, to fit into our daily lives without requiring a big change in our daily routines.
- Open, to allow a person that starts using a system to clearly know its purpose from the beginning.
- User-friendly, as a system is more effective when it is appealing and easy-to-use; however, recent approaches partially challenged this assumption, because even tools difficult to use could generate emotions and affection that influence both their usage and their persuasive power (cfr. Chap. 9).

The PSD model defines four categories of elements, or software features, based on what technology can do to persuade its users into changing their attitude or behavior: (1) primary task support; (2) dialogue support; (3) credibility support; (4) social support. Accordingly, different software features based on psychological theories can be chosen and implemented to reach the aim of supporting the user's primary activities, to facilitate the information flow between the computer and the user, to increase credibility about the presented information, or to leverage social influence.

In recent years, the PSD has been used both to better understand the impact of persuasive eHealth technology, as well as to evaluate which features are implemented in an eHealth solution, and their effects on adherence and outcome. It represents a promising field in the aim of changing behavior in the domain of health and well-being, but more studies are needed to get more insight into which features and subjective factors could predict the effectiveness of eHealth technology.

Once these aspects are better defined, it will be possible to define an optimal intervention for each individual, based on the selection of only those software features able to highly engage the subject. This could then be described by extending the P5 approach with a sixth "p" relevant to "persuasive," to describe the personalized process of defining a specific persuasive technology approach that could optimize the desired change in behavior, paving the way for a P6 approach conceptualization.

7 Conclusion

In this chapter, we have seen how eHealth could be based on a more accurate and systematic consideration of the psycho-cognitive uniqueness of individuals (and patients). Specifically, we have presented *persuasive technology* as a possible resource for designing technologies able to promote treatment adherence and healthy activities (e.g., behavioral change regarding lifestyle); however, we have to consider that medicine in general is a still evolving field. Although we have discussed that a consideration of psychological aspects is fundamental for the healthcare context to evolve toward patient centeredness, the research is still open to a complete understanding of the psycho-cognitive aspects to be included in the design and evaluation of technologies.

Future studies may focus on how technologies can help patients to perform decisions toward their healthcare process, by identifying the influence of biases and misconceptions that could lead patients toward making disadvantageous choices toward their own health management; such technologies could be used not only to aid medical practice (Lucchiari, Folgieri & Pravettoni, 2014), but also to empower patients (Woltmann et al., 2011); moreover, cognitive psychology would be included, in the form of theory-based prescriptions, in user-centered design approaches toward the development of health technologies, in order to take into consideration patients' mindset and cognitive abilities.

References

Abrams, M. A., Rita, S., Kurtz-Rossi, S., & Nielsen, G. (2012). *Always use teach-back!* Milano: Toolkit.

Adherence to long-term therapies. Evidence for action WHO. (2003). http://apps.who.int/medicinedocs/pdf/s4883e/s4883e.pdf

Bacigalupe, G., & Askari, S. F. (2013). E-Health innovations, collaboration, and healthcare disparities: Developing criteria for culturally competent evaluation. *Families, Systems, & Health, 31*(3), 248.

Bradford, D., & Palmer, A. F. (2016). *In strong hands: ehealth support for mental health carers. Poster session presented at the meeting of Computing and mental health.* San Jose, CA.

Britten, N., Pope, C., Halford, S., & Richeldi, L. (2016). What if we made stratified medicine work for patients? *Lancet Respiratory Medicine, 4*(1), 8–10.

Brownell, R., Kaminski, N., Woodruff, P. G., Bradford, W. Z., Richeldi, L., Martinez, F. J., & Collard, H. R. (2016). Precision medicine: The new frontier in idiopathic pulmonary fibrosis. [Review]. *American Journal of Respiratory and critical care medicine, 193*(11), 1213–1218. https://doi.org/10.1164/rccm.201601-0169CI.

Davis, T. C., Long, S. W., Jackson, R. H., Mayeaux, E. J., George, R. B., Murphy, P. W., & Crouch, M. A. (1993). Rapid estimate of adult literacy in medicine: A shortened screening instrument. *Family medicine, 25*(6), 391–395.

Eysenbach, G. (2008). Medicine 2.0: Social networking, collaboration, participation, apomediation, and openness. *Journal of medical Internet research, 10*(3).

Fogg, B. J. (2002). Persuasive technology: Using computers to change what we think and do. *Ubiquity, 2002*(December), 5.

Fumagalli, L. P., Radaelli, G., Lettieri, E., & Masella, C. (2015). Patient empowerment and its neighbours: Clarifying the boundaries and their mutual relationships. *Health Policy, 119*(3), 384–394.

Gorini, A., & Pravettoni, G. (2011). P5 medicine: a plus for a personalized approach to oncology. [Comment Letter Research Support, Non-U.S. Gov't]. *Nature Reviews Clinical Oncology, 8*(7), 444. https://doi.org/10.1038/nrclinonc.2010.227-c1.

Halcox, J. P., Wareham, K., Cardew, A., Gilmore, M., Barry, J. P., Phillips, C., & Gravenor, M. B. (2017). Assessment of remote heart rhythm sampling using the AliveCor heart monitor to screen for atrial fibrillation: the REHEARSE-AF study. *Circulation, 136*(19), 1784–1794.

Hood, L., & Friend, S. H. (2011). Predictive, personalized, preventive, participatory (P4) cancer medicine. [Review]. *Nature Reviews Clinical Oncology, 8*(3), 184–187. https://doi.org/10.1038/nrclinonc.2010.227.

Hughes, R. G., & Ortiz, E. (2005). Medication errors: why they happen, and how they can be prevented. *Journal of Infusion Nursing, 28*, 14–24.

Internet World Stats. (2018). https://www.internetworldstats.com/stats.htm

Joseph-Williams, N., Elwyn, G., & Edwards, A. (2014). Knowledge is not power for patients: A systematic review and thematic synthesis of patient-reported barriers and facilitators to shared decision making. *Patient Education and Counseling, 94*(3), 291–309.

Kay, M., Santos, J., & Takane, M. (2011). mHealth: New horizons for health through mobile technologies. *World Health Organization, 64*(7), 66–71.

Kelders, S. M., & van Gemert-Pijnen, J. E. L. (2013). Using log-data as a starting point to make eHealth more persuasive. In *International conference on persuasive technology* (pp. 99–109). Berlin/Heidelberg: Springer.

Kessels, R. P. (2003). Patients' memory for medical information. *Journal of the Royal Society of Medicine, 96*(5), 219–222.

Lucchiari, C., Folgieri, R., & Pravettoni, G. (2014). Fuzzy cognitive maps: a tool to improve diagnostic decisions. *Diagnosis, 1*(4), 289–293.

Mårtensson, L., & Hensing, G. (2012). Health literacy–a heterogeneous phenomenon: a literature review. *Scandinavian Journal of Caring Sciences, 26*(1), 151–160.

Mead, N., & Bower, P. (2000). Patient-centredness: A conceptual framework and review of the empirical literature. *Social Science & Medicine, 51*(7), 1087–1110.

MRC. (2017), from https://www.mrc.ac.uk/research/initiatives/stratified-medicine/

Norman, C. D., & Skinner, H. A. (2006). eHealth literacy: Essential skills for consumer health in a networked world. *Journal of Medical Internet Research, 8*(2).

Oinas-Kukkonen, H., & Harjumaa, M. (2018). Persuasive systems design: Key issues, process model and system features. In *Routledge handbook of policy design* (pp. 105–123). Routledge.

Parker, R. M., Baker, D. W., Williams, M. V., & Nurss, J. R. (1995). The test of functional health literacy in adults. *Journal of General Internal Medicine, 10*(10), 537–541.

Porter, K., Chen, Y., Estabrooks, P., Noel, L., Bailey, A., & Zoellner, J. (2016). Using teach-back to understand participant behavioral self-monitoring skills across health literacy level and behavioral condition. *Journal of Nutrition Education and Behavior, 48*(1), 20–26.

Potter, P. (1988). *Hippocrates Vol VI. Diseases, internal affections*. Cambridge, MA/London: Harvard University Press.

Pravettoni, G., & Gorini, A. (2011). A P5 cancer medicine approach: why personalized medicine cannot ignore psychology. [Research Support, Non-U.S. Gov't]. *Journal of Evaluation in Clinical Practice, 17*(4), 594–596. https://doi.org/10.1111/j.1365-2753.2011.01709.x.

Sørensen, K., Van den Broucke, S., Fullam, J., Doyle, G., Pelikan, J., Slonska, Z., & Brand, H. (2012). Health literacy and public health: A systematic review and integration of definitions and models. *BMC Public Health, 12*(1), 80.

Sykiotis, G. P., Kalliolias, G. D., & Papavassiliou, A. G. (2005). Pharmacogenetic principles in the Hippocratic writings. [Historical Article]. *Journal of Clinical Pharmacology, 45*(11), 1218–1220. https://doi.org/10.1177/0091270005281091.

Tang, P. C., & Lansky, D. (2005). The missing link: Bridging the patient–provider health information gap. *Health Affairs, 24*(5), 1290–1295.

Woltmann, E. M., Wilkniss, S. M., Teachout, A., McHugo, G. J., & Drake, R. E. (2011). Trial of an electronic decision support system to facilitate shared decision making in community mental health. *Psychiatric Services, 62*(1), 54–60.

Ziegelstein, R. C. (2015). Personomics. *JAMA Internal Medicine, 175*(6), 888–889. https://doi.org/10.1001/jamainternmed.2015.0861.

Part III
Important Aspects for P5 Technologies Development and Utilization

Chapter 8
Role of Next-Generation Sequencing Technologies in Personalized Medicine

Stefania Morganti, Paolo Tarantino, Emanuela Ferraro, Paolo D'Amico, Giulia Viale, Dario Trapani, Bruno Achutti Duso, and Giuseppe Curigliano

1 Historic Background of DNA Sequencing

Cancer is a genetic disease. Decades of research has led to this knowledge, showing that it is the accumulation of molecular alterations that is the key element of tumorigenesis, directing the acquisition of the malignant phenotype (Vogelstein et al. 2013). Genes involved in oncogenesis are classified in "oncogenes," whose activation is responsible for tumor transformation and oncosuppressors, whose inactivation leads to cellular proliferation. Mutations of oncogenes (gain of function) or oncosuppressors (loss of function) can be genetically inherited (germline), but they are mostly acquired and caused by DNA replication errors and/or exposure to carcinogens (Kinzler and Vogelstein 1996).

The understanding of cancer as a genetic disease, though multifactorial and non-Mendelian in the majority of the cases, has led researchers to focus on cancer cells genome, looking for the leading cause(s) of the pathological proliferation that ultimately cause cancer. The identification of specific driver genomic alterations allowed the development of targeted therapies, more effective and less toxic compared to standard chemotherapies. Trastuzumab (approved in 1998) and imatinib (approved in 2001) were the first two drugs to show the potential of targeted therapy, followed by many molecules nowadays approved for the treatment of several types of cancer (Fischer et al. 2003). Interestingly, the US Food and Drug Administration (FDA) granted an accelerated approval for imatinib for the dramatic sustained response of chronic myelocytic leukemia (CML) patients treated with the novel tailored approach (Johnson et al. 2003), in 2001; today, both imatinib and

S. Morganti · P. Tarantino · E. Ferraro · P. D'Amico · G. Viale · D. Trapani
B. A. Duso · G. Curigliano (✉)
Division of Early Drug Development for Innovative Therapy, IEO,
European Institute of Oncology IRCCS, Milan, Italy

Department of Oncology and Hemato-Oncology (DIPO), University of Milan, Milan, Italy
e-mail: giuseppe.curigliano@ieo.it

G. Pravettoni, S. Triberti (eds.), *P5 eHealth: An Agenda for the Health Technologies of the Future*, https://doi.org/10.1007/978-3-030-27994-3_8

trastuzumab are enlisted as "essential medicines" by the World Health Organization, for the treatment of CML and breast cancer, available as a generic and biosimilar, respectively.

Genetic testing soon became a standard in oncological care: in the 2000s we have started to stratify patients according to their tumor mutational profile, tailoring therapies according to the genetic signature. However, we only aimed genetic testing at those few mutations known to be targetable in each specific tumor type, thus limiting the information acquired in a strict disease-oriented manner. In order to better understand the relevance of cancer mutations across different tumour types and easier identify new actionable targets, a reference "normal" genome sequence was needed to compare with the abnormal ones. The Human Genome Project provided such a feature in 2003, thanks to an international effort lasting almost 15 years, the project was accomplished using the Sanger sequencing technique to determine the exact sequence of nucleotide base pairs of the human genome (Green et al. 2015). During the same years, researchers kept studying the basic mechanisms of cancer growth, identifying new oncogenes and oncosuppressors. With a complete human genome reference in hand, it finally became possible to confirm the pathogenic alterations and to discover new genetic variants linked to human diseases. Large-scale cancer sequencing projects, such as the American TCGA (The Cancer Genome Atlas) and the British Cancer Genome Project were born with this purpose, giving birth to the "genomic era" of cancer research, thus promoting the progressive evolution of sequencing methods: in 2004, 454 Life Sciences showcased a paralleled form of sequencing called pyrosequencing, decreasing sequencing expenses at six-fold compared with Sanger sequencing. This technological implementation led to the birth of the first of many NGS platforms, which allowed a faster and simpler sequencing by employing microscopic, spatially separated DNA templates to massively parallelize the capture of data. With such platforms in hand, it became possible to sequence all the coding exons of a genome (Whole Exome Sequencing, WES) and even a full genome (Whole Genome Sequencing, WGS) in a short time and at an affordable price, providing a huge amount of data. Analyzing and interpreting this data promises to be the challenge of the next decades (Fig. 8.1).

1.1 The NGS Revolution in the Context of Precision Medicine

Besides improving our understanding of cancer, NGS promoted the birth of a new way of treating cancer patients, which we today call Precision Medicine (PM). With this term, we refer to the suiting of medical therapy to the individual characteristics of each subject and its condition (cfr. Chap. 5). In cancer care, this means tailoring oncological treatments to each patient's features and each cancer genomic alterations. It is not a new concept, but the use of NGS and the consequent availability of large-scale human genome databases have created an opportunity for significant onward movement of this approach.

We have already moved from a One-size-fits-all Medicine to a progressive stratification of patients according to their disease subtype, clinical features, and bio-

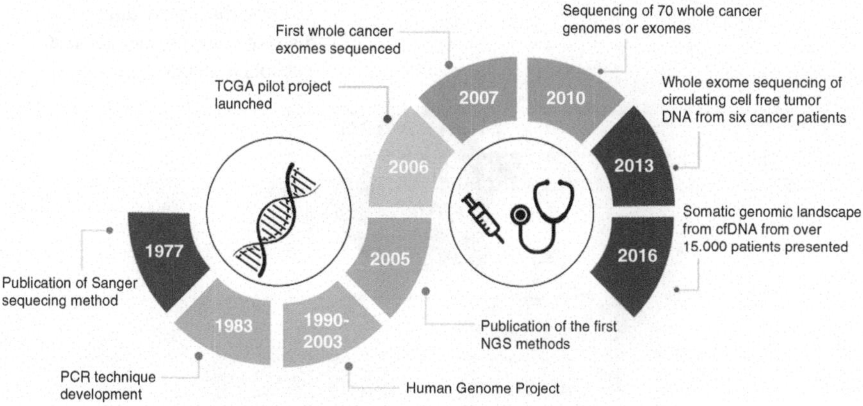

Fig. 8.1 Timeline of major achievements in sequencing technologies

markers (Stratified Medicine). NGS promises to lead the shift toward Precision Medicine, taking into account a wide set of patient features and the cancer mutational scenario to select the best therapeutic approach in oncological care (Shin et al. 2017) (Fig. 8.2).

PM in oncology involves identifying mutations in cancer genomes predicting response or resistance to therapies. In the pre-NGS era, Sanger sequencing and PCR (polymerase chain reaction)-based techniques allowed to obtain a limited amount of information on cancer mutational status; with NGS panels it is now possible instead to screen a broad set of genes in one comprehensive test, able to identify alterations even in the scarce biopsy tissue often available in the everyday practice. And in those frequent cases where collecting tissue for molecular testing is unsafe (e.g., brain, lung, peritoneal lesions), NGS allows to obtain extensive genetic information from simple blood draws (see "Liquid Biopsy" below). In fact, it is possible to obtain genetic material for sequencing from circulating tumor cells (CTCs) and circulating cell-free tumor DNA (ctDNA), which represents a unique instrument to capture the intratumoral heterogeneity, to identify prognostic and predictive factors and imminent resistance mechanisms (Ignatiadis and Dawson 2014). It was recently proposed to incorporate this instrument into cancer staging, shifting to a TNM-B cancer staging system to be assessed in the diagnosis of every cancer and at every successive stage of the disease (Yang et al. 2017).

2 Technical Aspects: From Sanger Sequencing to NGS

In 1977, Frederick Sanger and colleagues first developed a technique to sequence DNA (Sanger et al. 1977). Also known as "chain-termination method," it can be described as a DNA replication reaction during which the random incorporation of dideoxynucleotides (ddNTP) causes the termination of chain elongation. This generates DNA strands of various lengths that are later separated by electrophoresis.

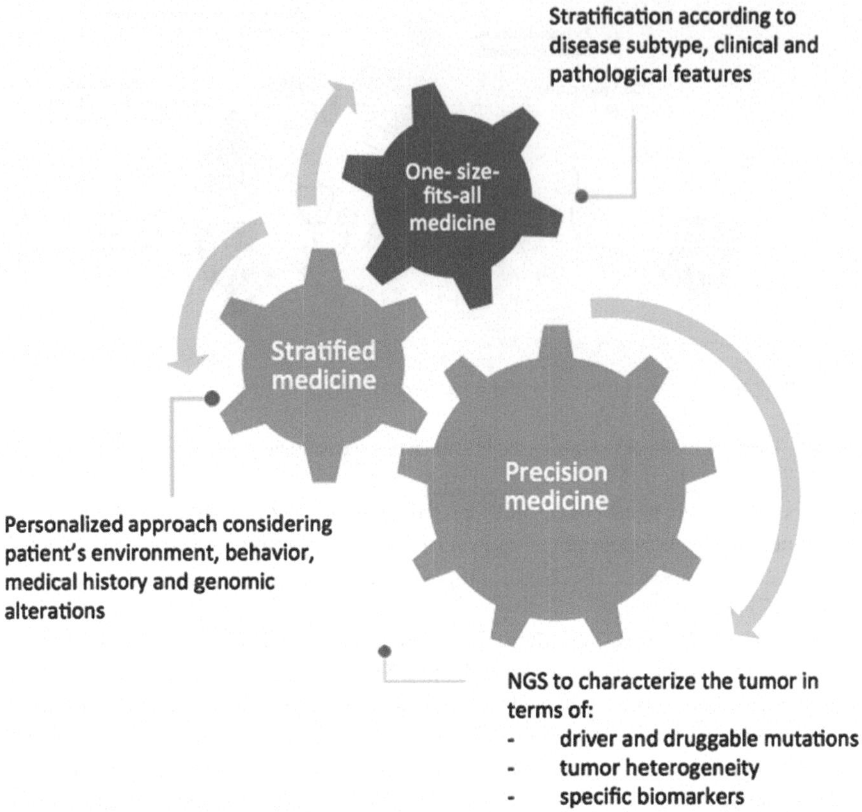

Fig. 8.2 Comprehensive approach in cancer care

Elements required for a classic chain-termination reaction are illustrated in Table 8.1.

The Sanger process is a very accurate sequencing method, giving high-quality sequence for relatively long fragments of DNA (up to 900 base pairs). On the other hand, it is a very expensive process with a low data output.

The need for simpler and faster sequencing processes led to the development of new technologies for DNA reading, collectively named "next-generation sequencing" (NGS). In 2005, the 454 Life Science launched on market the first NGS platform (Margulies et al. 2005), and since then many other companies developed NGS platforms that allow for high-throughput sequencing in a cost- and time-effective way.

Despite the platform used, every NGS process can be summarized in three phases: library preparation (± amplification), sequencing, and data analysis.

Table 8.1 Basic elements of a Sanger sequencing reaction

Table	A single-strand DNA sample that is previously amplified by PCR to generate many identical copies of a DNA sequence of interest.
DNA polymerase	The enzyme that sequentially adds nucleotides into the elongating chain. It catalyzes the reaction: dNTP (or ddNTP) + DNAn $\rightleftharpoons$ diphosphate + DNAn+1.
Primers	Short sequences of nucleotides (almost 20) that bind to the DNA template and act as a starter for the DNA polymerase.
Deoxynucleotides (dATP, dCTP, dGTP, dTTP)	Monomers that compose a DNA sequence. Each of them consists of a nitrogenous base, a deoxyribose sugar, and a phosphate group.
Dideoxynucleotides (ddATP, ddCTP, ddGTP, ddTTP)	ddNTP are special, artificial nucleotides analogous to dNTP, but lacking the –OH group at 3' carbon position. They act as chain-elongating inhibitors of DNA polymerase.
	To permit automate reading, ddNTP are usually labeled.

dNTP deoxynucleotides, *ddNTP* dideoxynucelotides, *PCR* polymerase chain reaction

2.1 Library Preparation and Amplification

The sequencing library is created by random fragmentation of a DNA template. Fragments are then linked to platform-specific adapters and amplified by PCR (polymerase chain reaction) or alternative techniques (solid-phase bridge amplification or rolling circle amplification).

2.2 Sequencing

NGS technology can be categorized into short- and long-read sequencing. The difference intuitively lies on read length: 100–600 bp for the first technique, up to 900 Kb for the second one.

Short-read sequencing approach is the most frequently used today—it is cheaper and has a higher accuracy. However, the short-read length limits its capability to resolve complex regions with repetitive or heterozygous sequences, for which a long-read technique is more suitable.

Illumina, Ion Torrent, 454 Life Science, and SOLiD are the major platforms created using a short-read technology. The first three platforms use a technique called sequencing "by synthesis," whereas the SOLiD system is based on sequencing "by ligation."

The MinION system, based on nanopore sequencing, and the PacBio sequencer, which uses a "Single Molecule, Real-Time (SMRT)" sequencing approach, represent instead the main long-read technologies available on the market. A technical comparison of all these NGS platforms is given in Table 8.2.

2.3 Data Analysis

The large amount of raw data generated is then inserted into bioinformatics workflows in order to convert these nucleotide sequences into meaningful biological results.

A typical NGS data analysis pipeline can be divided into four main operations: base calling, read alignment, variant identification (SNVs, indels, CNAs, SVs), and variant annotation. Table 8.3 briefly describes these steps.

3 NGS Methods: Genomics, Transcriptomics, and Epigenomics

3.1 Genomics

Next-generation sequencing was first applied to genomics research, mainly to detect variants in DNA sequence in terms of single nucleotide variations (SNVs), insertion-deletions (indels), structural variations (SVs), and copy number alterations (CNAs).

NGS methodology applied to an entire genome is called "whole genome sequencing," in which both coding and non-coding regions are sequenced. WGS generates huge amounts of data per sample, but usually low depth of coverage. A typical WGS experiment assures a 30X coverage, enough to detect most germline variants in human genome, but inadequate to identify all rare somatic mutations present in cancer genomes.

"Whole exome sequencing" is instead specifically designed to sequence only coding DNA. These regions are isolated before sequencing by an enrichment step, which targets only the exons inside the library of interest. By sequencing only 2% of a genome, a single region can be read many more times, ensuring a coverage of 100X with a cheaper and faster process. WES is therefore more suitable to analyze cancer genome; however, the capability to detect SVs and CNVs is much lower when excluding non-coding regions.

An even more selective genome analysis is given by "targeted sequencing," in which specific regions of interest are isolated and sequenced. Many gene panels have been designed specifically for this purpose, allowing to focus time and resources on selected genes usually sequenced with a 500–1000X coverage.

Table 8.2 Comparison between commercially available NGS platforms

Platform	Sequencing	Maximum read lenght (bp)	Reads per run	Run time	Maximum output	Error rate
First generation						
Sanger	NA	900	96	20 min–3 h	2.1 Mb	0.3%
Second generation						
454						
GS Junior+	Pyro	700	0.1 M	18 h	70 Mb	1% indels
GS FLX Titanium XL+	Pyro	700	1 M	23 h	700 Mb	1% indels
Illumina						
Hi Seq[a]	SBS	36 (SE)	Up to 4 B (SE)	<1–3.5 h (Hi Seq 3000/4000)	1500 Gb	0.1%
		125 (PE)	Up to 8 B (PE)	7 h – 6 d (Hi Seq 2500)		substitution
MiniSeq[b]	SBS	150 (PE)	25 M	4–24 h	7.5 Gb	<1%
						substitution
NextSeq 550[b]	SBS	75 (SE)	Up to 400 M (SE)	12–30 h	120 Gb	<1%
		150 (PE)	Up to 800 M (PE)			substitution
MiSeq (v3)	SBS	75 (PE)	25 M (PE)	4–55 h	15 Gb	0.1%
		300 (PE)				substitution
Hi SeqX[a]	SBS	150 (PE)	5.3-6 B	<3 d	1800 Gb	0.1%
						substitution
NovaSeq6000[c]	SBS	150 (PE)	20 B	36–44 h	6000 Gb	NA
Ion Torrent						
PGM	SBS	400 (SE)	400000–5.5 M	2.3–7.3 h	2 Gb	1% indels
Proton	SBS	Up to 200 (SE)	60–80 M	2–4 h	Up to 10 Gb	1% indels
S5	SBS	600 (SE)	2–130 M	2.5–4 h	25 Gb	1% indels
SOLiD (Sequencing by Oligonucleotide Ligation and Detection)						
5500xl	SBL	75 (SE)	~1.4 B	10 d	240 Gb	0.01%
		50 (PE)				A-T bias
Third generation						
PacBio (Pacific Bioscience)						
RS II	SMRT	>15000 (average)	Up to 55000	30 min–4 h	1 Gb	15% indels
Sequel	SMRT	30000 (average)	~400000	30 min–20 h	10 Gb	15%

(continued)

Table 8.2 (continued)

Platform	Sequencing	Maximum read lenght (bp)	Reads per run	Run time	Maximum output	Error rate
Oxford Nanopore						
MinION	SMRT	Up to 900 kb	Up to 1 M	Up to 48 h	20 Gb	5–10%

A-T adenine-thymine, *B* billion, *bp* base pairs, *d* days, *Gb* gigabase pairs, *h* hours, *indels* insertions-deletions, *Kb* kilobase pairs, *M* million, *Mb* megabase pairs, *min* minutes, *NA* not applicable, *PE* pair-end, *Pyro* pyrosequencing, *SBL* sequencing by ligation, *SBS* sequencing by synthesis, *SE* single-end, *SMRT* single-molecule-real-time
[a]Dual flow cells; [b]high output; [c]dual S2 flow cells

Table 8.3 Basic steps of NGS data processing

Base calling	Signals provided during sequencing are translated into a sequence of bases, removing the noisy signals.
Read alignment	DNA of the sequenced sample is compared/aligned to a reference genome. Given that NGS generally produces millions of short reads, each read needs to find the corresponding part on reference genome.
Variant identification/ calling	Variants from sequence data are identified in this step. Four main classes of sequence variants exist (SNVs, indels, CNAs, and SVs), each requiring a different computational approach for sensitive and specific identification.
Variant annotation	Real variants are distinguished from sequencing artefacts, trying to identify which ones are potentially pathogenic and have a real clinical value.

SNVs single nucleotide variations, *indels* insertion/deletion, *CNAs* copy number alterations, *SVs* structure variants

3.2 Transcriptomics

The transcriptome can be defined as "the complete set of transcripts in a cell or a population of cells for a specific developmental stage or physiological condition" (Wang et al. 2009). Transcriptomics studies have a pivotal role in cancer research, providing a unique focus of what happens in neoplastic cells after DNA transcription.

RNA-sequencing (RNA-seq) is a relatively new application of NGS, which is gradually replacing microarrays as favorite technology for transcripts analysis. Differently from arrays, RNA-seq is not designed as a targeted test and does not require species- or transcript-specific probes. It can be used both to quantify gene expression and to detect novel transcripts, gene fusions, SNV, and indels at the same time.

Besides gene expression analysis, NGS has also been applied to small non-coding RNA (ncRNA) discovery and profiling through dedicated small RNA-seq platforms. Small non-coding RNAs are short sequences of nucleotides (≈20 bp) not translated into proteins. Several classes of small ncRNA exist, like transfer RNA (tRNA), ribosomal RNA (rRNA), microRNA (miRNA), small interfering RNA (siRNA), and Piwi-interacting RNA (piRNA). Between them, miRNA and siRNA are of major interest to transcriptomic research in oncology because of their role in gene expression regulation of cancer cells (Gomes et al. 2013). Through a cellular process called RNA interference (RNAi), both miRNA and siRNA interact with the so-called RNA-induced silencing complex (RISC) to block and silence target mRNAs.

This powerful gene-silencing process is object of study also from a therapeutic point of view. RNA-based therapeutics represents a new class of anticancer drugs, inhibiting molecules targets that were inaccessible until now. None of these drugs is approved by FDA to date, but many are currently under investigation in clinical trials (Barata et al. 2016).

3.3 Epigenomics

The term epigenetics refers to "the study of changes in gene function that are mitotically and/or meiotically heritable and that do not entail a change in DNA sequence" (Wu and Morris 2001). DNA methylation, histone-modification, and altered DNA–protein interactions are three major epigenetic alterations involved in cancer development and progression.

In the past years, epigenomics studies were essentially conducted through microarrays technologies. The arrival of NGS signed a paradigm shift in this field, dramatically increasing the chance to survey epigenetic markers genomewide with high-throughput data output at single nucleotide resolution. Methylation sequencing (or bisulfite sequencing) (Lister et al. 2008) and ChIP-seq (Chromatin Immunoprecipitation Sequencing) (Barski et al. 2007) are the NGS-based assays commonly employed for epigenetics studies.

4 NGS Applications for a Personalized Oncology

4.1 Detection of Driver Alterations and Resistance

The availability of next-generation sequencing technologies had literally revolutionized the comprehension of cancer biology during the last decades. Massive genome sequencing of thousands of tumors from all major cancer types has become feasible, leading to identification and classification of many genetic and epigenetic alterations potentially involved in tumorigenesis.

By the time a cancer is diagnosed, it comprises billions of these genomic alterations. Some are responsible for malignant transformation, others are acquired along the way. The pivotal work of Greenman and coworkers defined these two categories of mutations as "driver" and "passenger" (Greenman et al. 2007). The term "driver" is reserved for somatic mutations that, directly or indirectly, confer a selective growth advantage to malignancies bearing them. The term "passenger" is instead referred to alterations that arise in somatic cancer genome during the progression of a tumor, but do not contribute to its growth.

Detection of driver alterations that results in oncogene addiction is currently the primary application of NGS in oncology research and discriminating between driver and passenger alterations is a challenge point of translational research. Several statistical and computational techniques to characterize these mutations have been described, including variant effect prediction, recurrence/frequency assessment, and pathway/network analysis. These techniques provide alternative strategies to filter the long list of somatic mutations, thus identifying an enriched subset of subclonal carriers who may undergo further functional validation (Gonzalez-Perez et al. 2013; Raphael et al. 2014; Ding et al. 2014). Given that driver mutations are responsible for oncogenic addiction, any targeted therapy must be based on their identification. The implementation of this "lock-and-key" model led to the approval of several specific biologic agents, targeting specific driver alterations in different cancer types.

Here we present the example of NGS application in clinical practice for identification of driver and resistance mutations in lung cancer, breast cancer, and cancer of unknown primary origin.

4.1.1 Lung Cancer

Lung cancer represents, by far, the disease in which pathways of oncogenic addiction have been characterized the most. There are, on average, more than 300 nonsynonymous mutations per lung cancer, but only a minority of these genes can promote tumorigenesis, resulting in driver mutations. Large-scale genomic studies have recognized a variety of potential therapeutic targeting, including:

- Established targets: EGFR, ALK, ROS-1, BRAF
- Emergent target: MET, RET, NTRK, HER2, PI3KCA, AKT1, MAP 3K1, FGFR, DDR2
- Elusive targets: KRAS, TP53

International guidelines recommend molecular testing for these established targets in everyday clinical practice.

Detection of EGFR and BRAF mutations are classically carried out using RT-PCR (Real Time-PCR) or Sanger sequencing, whereas ALK and ROS1 rearrangements are identified through FISH (fluorescence in situ hybridization) or IHC (immunohistochemistry) methods. In recent years, NGS panels implementation is gradually replacing these techniques in clinical laboratories, allowing the analysis of several genes at the same time. The last MAP (Molecular Analysis for Personalised Therapy) consensus (Swanton et al. 2016) recommends the use of NGS panels in the context of clinical trials. For non-small-cell lung cancer (NSCLC), at least 20 genes should be tested in molecular screening programs to drive patients onto therapeutic trials (EGFR, BRAF, HER2, KRAS, PI3KCA, NTKR, ALK, MET, AKT1, BRCA1/BRCA2, HRAS, NRAS; rearrangement status of ALK, ROS1, NTRK;

amplification of RET, MET, and EGFR; aberrations (mutations or amplifications) in FGFR1/2/3, NOTCH1/NOTCH2).

Profiling of EGFR, ALK, ROS1, and BRAF defines as many "subtypes" of NSCLC, for which specific algorithm of treatment exists. Activating EGFR mutations in the tyrosine kinase (TK) domain of the EGFR gene, most frequently exon 19 deletion mutations and the single-point substitution mutation L858R in exon 21, are predictive for response to the EGFR TK Inhibitors (EGFR-TKIs) gefitinib, erlotinib, afatinib, osimertinib, and dacomitinib. ALK rearrangement-positive NSCLC are instead candidate to frontline therapy with ALK-inhibitors alectinib, crizotinib, or ceritinib. The last two of them are also the referred targeted drugs for ROS1-rearranged NSCLC, whereas cancers positive for BRAF V600E can receive the combination dabrafenib-trametinib (www.nccn.org/professionals/physician_gls/pdf/nscl.pdf).

Unfortunately, almost all patients treated with targeted therapies develop secondary resistance. NGS can be useful to identify the implicated mechanisms of resistance and to aid on following treatment choices. For instance, T790M mutation has been found in almost 50% of patients that progress during treatment with first- and second-generation EGFR-TKIs. This finding led to the development of osimertinib, a third-generation EGFR TKI that inhibits T790M as well as the common activating mutations. The AURA 3 trial (Mok et al. 2017) demonstrated the great superiority of osimertinib to platinum-based chemotherapy in EGFR-TKIs pretreated patients with T790M mutation, reporting a PFS of 10.1 months in osimetinib group versus 4.4 months in the control group. The introduction of osimertinib has allowed prolonging as far as possible the chemo-free interval in EGFR-positive population.

Interestingly, the T790M mutation was documented using the Cobas EGFR Mutation Test v2 on ctDNA on blood and urine samples. Osimertinib is currently approved only for T790M-positive NSCLC, and this mutation can be indifferently assessed on tissue sample or liquid biopsy. In this common clinical scenario, preferring blood- over tissue-sampling is clinical practice.

4.1.2 Breast Cancer

The estrogen receptor (ER) and the HER2 signaling pathways are the dominant drivers of oncogenesis in breast cancer. The available arsenal of hormonal agents and anti-HER2 drugs has dramatically changed the natural history of metastatic breast cancer (MBC) during last decades, achieving a twofold increase in 5-year relative survival rate (Mariotto et al., 2017).

Unfortunately, ER-expression and/or HER2-amplification can well predict but are not secure guarantee of response to targeted therapy with endocrine therapy and HER2-signaling blocking agents. Many patients are resistant *ab initio* (de novo resistance), whereas others become resistant after an initial phase of therapeutic efficacy (acquired/secondary resistance).

ESR1 mutations in ER-positive breast cancer is a recognized cause of resistance to endocrine therapy, more commonly as acquired resistance. First described in cell models in 1996 (Weis et al. 1996), ESR1 mutations were found to confer ER constitutive activation and resistance to endocrine agents. Nevertheless, these alterations were rarely found in subsequent studies (0.5% of cases), and their potential role remained underappreciated for several years (Koboldt et al. 2012).

With NGS technology applications, several studies renewed interest in ESR1 mutations by demonstrating high prevalence in ER-positive MBC after aromatase inhibitor (AIs) therapy, suggesting a role in the endocrine resistance, both as predictive and prognostic biomarker (Schiavon et al. 2015; Jeselsohn et al. 2014; Merenbakh-Lamin et al. 2013; Robinson et al. 2013).

The SOFEA trial compared exemestane alone with fulvestrant-containing regimens (fulvestrant+anastrozole or fulvestrant +placebo) in patients with MBC pretreated with AIs (Johnston et al., 2013). In a retrospective analysis of this trial, detection of ESR1 mutations (39% of patients) correlated with an improved PFS after taking fulvestrant compared with exemestane, whereas wild-type patients had similar outcomes with both treatments (Fribbens et al. 2016).

Additionally, a retrospective analysis of the BOLERO-2 trial, evaluating the benefit of incorporating everolimus to AI therapy, showed longer PFS with everolimus only in the subgroup of patients harboring D538G ESR1 mutations (21.1%), with similar outcomes when compared to wild-type patients. This benefit was not observed for patients with Y537S mutation (alone or with D538G mutation). Despite the treatment arm, all patients ESR1-mutated had a worse overall survival (OS). The authors concluded that ESR1 mutations are not predictive of benefit with everolimus, but ESR1 keeps a negative prognostic value (Chandarlapaty et al. 2016).

In the PALOMA3 trial, pre- and postmenopausal patients failing a prior ET within 12 months in the adjuvant and 1 month in the metastatic setting were randomized to fulvestrant plus palbociclib or fulvestrant and placebo (Cristofanilli et al. 2016). ESR1 mutations were detected in 25% of patients, at baseline, as a finding related to the endocrine resistance mechanism. A significant PFS benefit was reported for patients treated with fulvestrant/palbociclib versus patients receiving fulvestrant alone, and this benefit was maintained in patients harboring an ESR1 mutation. This evidence confirms a conserved selective sensitivity to fulvestrant for ESR1-mutant cancers, even if these mutations are commonly associated with a worse prognosis (Turner et al. 2016). In conclusion, the suggestion is to select the combination fulvestrant +/- palbociclib over AIs when ESR1 mutations are detected.

Prospective trials are needed to understand if ESR1 mutations analysis could impact on treatment choice and final outcome of ER-positive MBC. Specific inhibitors are under investigation like AZD9496, in a refined targeted approach to endocrine therapy (Hamilton et al. 2018).

4.1.3 Carcinoma of Unknown Primary Site

Management of carcinoma of unknown primary (CUP) site is another field that made considerable steps forward since NGS availability. CUP accounts for 3–5% of all malignancies, the seventh for incidence and the fourth cause of cancer death

(Massard et al. 2011). ESMO guidelines recommend a platinum-based regimen for the majority of CUP patients (85–90% of cases), defined as "poor-risk" subset because of lacking any clinico-pathological features that provide a favorable outcome. Their prognosis is dismal despite chemotherapy (median OS of 9 months) (Fizazi et al. 2015).

Thanks to NGS profiling, CUP management has radically changed. First of all, it has been shown that gene expression profiling can predict the tissue of origin and consequently allow treatment optimization, in a histology-oriented approach. A prospective trial conducted by Hainsworth and colleagues at the Sarah Cannon Research Institute found that the primary tissue can be predicted in 98% of cases. Patients in this trial were subsequently treated with a site-specific regimen, reaching a median survival of 12.5 months (Hainsworth et al. 2012). Considering the modest benefit achieved with a platinum-based empiric regimen, the identification of the putative primary may substantially change the management and outcome of patients with CUP, particularly if a tumor more responsive to the best site-specific therapy is recognized.

Detection of actionable mutation is another promising application of the genome sequencing for a molecular-oriented approach to CUP management. Performing a sequencing panel encompassing 410 cancer-associated genes (the MSK-IMPACT panel), Varghese et al. analyzed 150 tissue samples of CUP. A targetable genomic alteration was found in 30% of cases (45 patients), and 10% of them (13 patients) received a targeted drug. The most common putative driver alterations detected were: ERBB2 amplification, BRAF V600E mutation, and PIK3CA mutations (Varghese et al. 2017).

"CUPISCO" is a randomized, phase II study designed to compare efficacy and safety of targeted therapy or immunotherapy versus platinum-based chemotherapy in CUP (NCT03498521). After three cycles of platinum-based induction CT, patients are randomized 3:1 to targeted therapy/immunotherapy or chemotherapy. A comprehensive genomic profiling is performed on all patients enrolled before receiving the induction CT, allowing a subsequent choice of the best targeted therapy in the experimental arm. This trial is actually recruiting and the first results are expected in 2022. If positive, their results could dramatically change the management of CUP in everyday clinical practice.

4.2 Biomarkers

In 1998, the National Institutes of Health Biomarkers Definitions Working Group defined a biomarker as "a characteristic that is objectively measured and evaluated as an indicator of normal biological processes, pathogenic processes, or pharmacologic responses to a therapeutic intervention" (Atkinson et al. 2001). A biomarker has a "prognostic" value when it gives information about disease outcome irrespective of treatment, whereas a "predictive" biomarker indicates the likely benefit from a specific treatment.

In the era of targeted therapy, predictive biomarkers and related targeted drugs are commonly validated and approved in parallel. HER2 amplification/trastuzumab in breast cancer, BCR-ABL translocation/imatinib in chronic myeloid leukemia, EGFR mutation/EGFR TKI in NSCLC, and BRAF mutation/melanoma are only few examples of "predictive biomarker/targeted drug" pairs that commonly guide the therapeutic choice.

Beside the well-known biomarkers for cancer treatment response prediction, relatively new and more complex models are emerging. Microsatellite instability (MSI), homologous recombination deficiency (HRD), and tumor mutation burden (TMB) have the most robust data so far and will probably soon impact on clinical practice as predictive of response to DNA-disrupting agents, DNA repair targeting compounds, and immunotherapy.

4.2.1 Homologous Recombination Deficiency

Homologous recombination (HR) is a genetic recombination mechanism essential for repair of DNA double-strand breaks (DSBs) (Jasin and Rothstein 2013; Szostak et al. 1983). BRCA1 and BRCA2 genes are essential components of HR-mediated DNA repair, and mutations of these genes cause HR pathway failure (Moynahan et al. 1999; Moynahan et al. 2001). In HR-deficient cells, other mechanism of DNA repair must take over, such as non-homologous end joining (NHEJ) or base-excision repair (BER) (Hustedt and Durocher 2017). Specific agents, like poly-(ADP ribose) polymerase (PARP) inhibitors, have been designed to target these alternative pathways (Fong et al. 2009; Robson et al. 2017; Swisher et al. 2017). This therapeutic strategy, called "synthetic lethality," sentences HR-deficient cells to die by apoptosis.

The singularity of HRD as predictive biomarker lies on its complexity. BRCA1/2 are only two of many proteins involved in this pathway, and all of these need to be analyzed in parallel to make HRD a reliable biomarker. Many panels based on NGS sequencing are currently available to test HRD in different cancers, providing a quantitative score that reveals if the HR pattern is impaired or not (O'Kane et al. 2017).

4.2.2 Microsatellite Instability

Microsatellite instability refers to hypermutability of short nucleotide sequences tandemly repeated (microsatellites) (Thibodeau et al. 1993). This condition is essentially due to impairment of DNA mismatch repair (MMR) pathway, because of mutation of MMR genes (e.g., MLH1, MSH2, MSH3, MSH6, and PMS2).

MSI is observed in 15% of sporadic colorectal tumors (Vilar Gruber 2010), and has been reported in tumors of endometrium, ovaries, urothelium, stomach, small intestine, hepatobiliary tract, brain, and skin. If instead a germline mutation is found, the MSI phenotype identifies a genetic disease called "hereditary non-polyposis colorectal cancer" (HNPCC), or Lynch syndrome (Lynch et al. 1993).

A potential role of MSI as predictive biomarker has recently been investigated, following the evidences that high levels of MSI seem to predict a good response to immune-checkpoint inhibitors (ICPI), whereas MSI stable tends not to (Le et al. 2017). This result led to the FDA approval of pembrolizumab for MSI-H cancers in May 2017, the first tumor-agnostic drug approval in history.

MS instability is usually analyzed through PCR and IHC assays. Nevertheless, dedicated NGS panels have been recently implemented, showing feasibility and reliability if compared to "old" techniques (Vanderwalde et al. 2018). The main advantages of NGS methodology over IHC and PCR are the unnecessity of normal tissue (unlike PCR), a quantitative result (instead of IHC, which is a qualitative test) and obviously the availability of many additional information for a therapy personalization at its best.

4.2.3 Tumor Mutational Burden

Tumor mutational burden is defined as the number of somatic mutations within the coding region of a tumor genome. A high mutational load is typically found in tumor associated to environmental DNA damage, like lung cancer (i.e., tobacco smoking, environmental pollution) or melanoma (i.e., sun exposure) (Chalmers et al. 2017).

TMB has recently been identified as predictive biomarker of immunotherapy efficacy. The rationale lies in the principle of immunotherapy itself: a TMB correlates with expression of multiple neoantigens by cancer cells, and consequently to potential efficacy of ICPI in reactivating immunity against cancer cells.

Major evidences about a role of TMB as predictive biomarker of response to ICPI come from retrospective analysis of different studies, including melanoma, NSCLC, and urothelial cancer (Rosenberg et al. 2016; Rizvi et al. 2015; Snyder et al. 2014). A prospective validation in phase III trials is awaited; however, early phase trials suggest a predictive role for TMB. Both in NSCLC and SCLC, the first-line combination therapy nivolumab + ipilimimab has shown to be more effective in patients with high TMB, as respectively outlined in Checkmate 227 (Hellmann et al. 2018a, b) and 032 (Hellmann et al. 2018a, b) trials. Similar evidences come from trials with atezolizumab in first- (B-F1RST study (Velcheti et al. 2018) and second-line (POPLAR and OAK trials (Gandara et al. 2017) treatment for NSCLC. Quantification of TMB was classically carried out through whole exome sequencing. This approach is accurate, but expensive and not suitable for routine use in clinical practice. For this reason, major biotechnology companies have designed specific targeted panels to quantify TMB in a simple and cost-effective way. Many independent trials have already proved their reliability if compared to WES (Johnson et al. 2016). Prospective trials are now necessary to validate their implementation in clinical practice to identify which patients are more likely to respond to immunotherapy.

4.3 *Liquid Biopsy*

Liquid biopsies are noninvasive blood tests that detect circulating tumor cells (CTCs) and fragments of tumor DNA (cell-free tumor DNA – ctDNA) released into the bloodstream from the primary tumor and from metastatic sites.

Collection of fluid instead of classic tissue sample is gradually spreading from research laboratories to clinical practice. A liquid biopsy consists of a simple blood sampling, overcoming the issues related to the feasibility of invasive biopsy procedures. For the same reason it can be repeated many times without risks or side effects, providing a picture of tumor evolution over time. Finally, analysis of ctDNA may allow a better representation of tumor heterogeneity, possibly detecting different clones at once. Many potential applications of liquid biopsy are object of ongoing clinical trials. The most promising are briefly presented below.

4.3.1 Early Diagnosis of Primary Disease

Early detection of cancer through a validated screening assay is probably the most ambitious purpose of liquid biopsy. Like every screening test, high sensitivity, specificity, and cost-effectiveness are essential requirements. Despite recent development of very sensitive technologies, a reliable test for early cancer detection remains a challenge.

Cohen et al. (2018) launched very recently the CancerSEEK panel, developed for detection of the eight most common cancers (ovary, liver, stomach, pancreas, esophagus, colorectum, lung, and breast). This method combines the evaluation of eight blood biomarkers with sequencing of 16 cancer-related genes from ctDNA. On a sample of 1005 individuals with clinically detected non-metastatic cancers, the authors reported a median sensitivity of 70% (ranging from 98% in ovarian cancers to 33% in breast cancers), with a specificity ≥99%. Despite these encouraging results, some limitations to this study must be noted. Firstly, the experimental cohort was composed by patients with clinically detected cancers. In a real-world screening population most individuals would have less advanced disease, probably determining a minor test sensitivity. Secondly, the control cohort included only health individuals, without all the comorbidities that could augment the number of false positive results.

4.3.2 Early Detection of Relapse

Several studies have demonstrated that CTCs detection is associated with unfavorable prognosis in various types of solid tumors, in particular for early-stage diseases.

Early breast cancer (EBC) is the setting for which more evidences exist. The largest trial realized so far has been published by Rack and colleagues in 2014

(Rack et al. 2014). The authors used the CellSearch System to analyze CTCs in patients with EBC: 2026 women were tested before adjuvant CT and 1492 after the treatment. CTCs detection before CT was associated with poor outcome both in terms of disease-free survival and overall survival. The persistence of CTCs after receiving adjuvant CT was analogously linked to a negative prognosis.

Beside breast cancer, CTCs count has been evaluated as prognostic marker for metastatic relapse in many other tumor types, like colorectal (Yokobori et al. 2013), bladder (Rink et al. 2012), liver (Schulze et al. 2013), head and neck (Gröbe et al. 2014), and testicular germ cell tumors (Nastaly et al. 2014).

Cell-free tumor DNA profiling has been similarly performed to assess its value in predicting metastatic relapse. In two different studies published in 2015, ctDNA was serially assessed for earlier detection of metastasis in patients with EBC. In both cases, mutation tracking in serial samples has been shown to accurately predict metastatic relapse, in several instances months before clinical relapse (8–11 months on average) (Olsson et al. 2015; Garcia-Murillas et al. 2015). Reinert et al. (2016) conducted a similar trial on patients with early colorectal cancer, with analogous final evidences: using an NGS approach on ctDNA it was possible to detect metastatic recurrence with a 10 months' lead time compared to conventional follow-up.

Taken together, these evidences suggest that implementation of liquid biopsy for screening of patients with high risk, early-stage cancer may create a therapeutic window for interventions before the development of clinical metastasis.

4.3.3 Detection of Driver/Resistance Mutations and Real-Time Monitoring of Therapies

As previously mentioned, detection of driver- and resistance mutations is a key application of NGS. DNA profiling is performed on a tissue sample from a biopsy or a surgical specimen, usually from the primary tumor and sometimes from a metastatic site. These samples are then archived in pathological labs, always available for additional analysis. Nevertheless, they may represent a "static" picture unable to reflect the temporal evolution under drug pressure. Moreover, metastatic relapse frequently happens several years after primary tumor resection, and the information obtained from that specimen might be outdated. Serial tissue biopsies of both primary tumors and metastatic sites are unfeasible in clinical practice. On the contrary, liquid biopsy allows repeated analyses over the course of treatment, providing a dynamic and reliable picture of tumor genome that can be used for monitoring therapies in real time.

Treatment choice in metastatic breast cancer is determined by ER-expression and HER2-amplification. ER-positive MBCs are eligible for hormonal treatment; that is, commonly continued until development of resistance and disease progression. A common cause of acquired resistance to endocrine therapy is tumor heterogeneity: patients with ER-positive BC can harbor ER-negative CTCs, as demonstrated by Paoletti et al. (2015).

Mutation of ER itself is a common cause of resistance. Chu and coworkers proved that somatic mutations in the ER gene (ESR1) can be readily identified in ctDNA, and they correlate with failure of endocrine therapy (Chu et al. 2016). Liquid biopsy has been also successfully applied for analysis of ESR1 methylation, known to be responsible for epigenetic silencing of ESR1 (ER downregulation) and development of secondary endocrine resistance (Mastoraki et al. 2018).

The HER2 oncogene is another key target in MBC treatment. Also, for HER2 status a discrepancy between CTCs and primary tumors has been found in up to 30% of cases (Fehm et al. 2010). This evidence inspired the development of dedicated interventional trials, where patients HER2-negative at primary assessment can receive anti-HER2 agents on the basis of HER2-status on CTCs (DETECT III study—NCT01619111, Treat CTC trial—NCT01548677). In colorectal cancer, NRAS, KRAS, and BRAF status are essential requirements for therapy optimization. Many studies have reported a high level of concordance between mutational analysis on tissue samples and ctDNA (Mouliere et al. 2013; Siravegna et al. 2015). Moreover, liquid biopsy has shown to provide a better picture of tumor heterogeneity, detecting RAS mutation not found on tissue sample (Siravegna et al. 2015).

Mutational analysis of KRAS status during treatment with anti-EGFR can also predict disease progression several months before radiologic assessment (Misale et al. 2012). Longitudinal ctDNA profiling has even demonstrated that these mutant KRAS clones decline following anti-EGFR withdrawal, indicating that clonal evolution is a continuous process (Siravegna et al. 2015).

Lung cancer is the prototype of therapy personalization based on mutational status. Once again, liquid sequencing has proved to be a reliable surrogate of tissue biopsy (Kuang et al. 2009; Taniguchi et al. 2011; Nakamura et al. 2012; Douillard et al. 2014; Reck et al. 2016). On June 1, 2016, FDA approved "Cobas EGFR Mutation Test v2" as first liquid biopsy test available in clinical practice. It is licensed for the detection of exon 19 deletions or exon 21 substitutions in EGFR gene. If negative, guidelines recommend a routine test using tissue sample to be performed (www.nccn.org/professionals/physician_gls/pdf/nscl.pdf).

EGFR profiling through liquid biopsy is a useful tool also during treatment with TKIs, allowing for detection of EGFR mutations responsible for therapy resistance. Oxnard et al. analyzed plasma ctDNA in 9 patients with EGFR-mutated NSCLC treated with erlotinib. All patients were negative for mutation T790M before starting treatment, but in 2/3 of them serial ctDNA profiling showed an increasing in T790M EGFR mutant levels up to 16 weeks before radiologic progression, anticipating the clinical–radiological progression (Oxnard et al. 2014).

Androgen blockade represents the cornerstone for treatment of prostate cancer. Unfortunately, progression to castration-resistant prostate cancer (CRPC) occurs virtually in all patients. Genomic and transcriptomic alterations of androgen receptor, essentially in terms of AR amplification and AR splice variants, are primarily responsible for progression to castration resistance.

AR-v7 is a splicing variant of AR, a truncated form of the receptor that is constitutively active because of lacking the ligand-binding domain. When detected, it is responsible not only for resistance to classical first-line androgen-deprivation therapy, but also to second-generation anti-androgen agents commonly applied in CRPC (i.e., enzalutamide and abiraterone). AR-v7 is commonly tested analyzing mRNA from CTCs (Antonarakis et al. 2014).

A recent clinical audit published by Johns Hopkins University has confirmed the potentiality of AR-v7 as predictive biomarker, revealing that its knowledge can influence the clinical decision making in 53% of patients (Markowski et al. 2017). Nevertheless, (it must be pointed out that) the last St. Gallen prostate cancer conference has discouraged a routine use of AR-v7 testing in clinical practice, mainly because only single-center experiences are available, and a prospective, external validation is still lacking (Gillessen et al. 2018). Moreover, AR-V7 positivity is 3% (Scher et al. 2016) in patients naive to abiraterone, enzalutamide, or taxane exposure, increasing only after progression on second-generation anti-androgen agents (19–39%) (Antonarakis et al. 2014). For this reason, the panel concluded for its limited value both in first-line setting, for its low-rate detection, and in second line, where chemotherapy is already the treatment of choice.

4.3.4 Characterization of Tumor Heterogeneity

Genetic diversity exists between individuals with the same tumor type (intertumor heterogeneity), but also within a single tumor (intratumor heterogeneity). Intratumor heterogeneity (ITH) is both spatial, comprising different subclones inside a unique lesion and in distinct sites, and temporal, emerging during the evolution of a malignancy.

The "trunk and branch" model is commonly used to represent ITH. Into the trunk are found driver somatic alterations that arise very early during the natural history of a tumor. Since indispensable for neoplastic growth, they are detectable in every subclone and tumor region. Conversely, subclonal mutations that occur later during cancer evolution are not homogeneously localized, but present in only a subset of cancer cells. They make up the branches of the tree (Yap et al. 2012).

In a pivotal paper published on Science almost 40 years ago, Peter Nowell firstly postulated this theory of cancer as a process of clonal evolution, in which successive rounds of clonal selection give rise to tumor heterogeneity (Nowell 1976). However, this theory could find a clinical application outside the preclinical experiments only years later, with the emergence of NGS techniques. Serial extensive tissue sampling of both primary and metastatic lesions is unfeasible in clinical practice, and sampling bias may occur because only limited geographical regions are analyzed.

The advent of next-generation sequencing has dramatically improved our understanding over tumor evolution, starting to resolve the complexity of ITH at single-nucleotide level. Given that ctDNA is a reliable noninvasive surrogate for tissue biopsies, massive parallel sequencing of ctDNA is likely to be the most powerful tool available to investigate ITH.

In a proof-of-concept study, De Mattos-Arruda et al. sequenced the genome of a primary cancer, a liver metastasis, and plasma ctDNA from a single patient with synchronous ER+/HER2- metastatic breast cancer. Using a targeted panel of 300 cancer genes, they found in ctDNA all the mutations present in the primary tumor and/or the liver metastasis. Conversely, not all mutated genes detected in the metastasis were reliably identified in the primary. The authors successfully proved that ctDNA sequencing is clearly a powerful tool for heterogeneity investigation, providing an accurate representation of the complete repertoire of mutations detected in all tumor sites (De Mattos-Arruda et al. 2014).

Many other studies conducted on different cancer types outlined analogous results (Siravegna et al. 2015; Landau et al. 2013; Lebofsky et al. 2015). Based on this assumption, ongoing trials have been conceived to monitor disease evolution prospectively, from early-stage diagnosis through the different stages of tumor progression and metastatic spreading.

The TRACERx is a pioneering project in this research field. Consisting of four parallel observational studies (lung, renal, melanoma, prostate), it is built on the ambitious aim of understanding the relationships between cancer genomic evolution in metastases, immune evasion, adaptation, and clinical outcome (http://tracerx.co.uk/).

4.3.5 CTCs and ctDNA Analysis

CTCs and ctDNA are cancer biomarkers with complementary roles. Outlining different information, they can be more or less useful with regard to specific research needs and clinical contexts. CTCs can be isolated by several methods, using physical, immunologic, molecular, or functional assays [98]. Several platforms for CTCs detection are commercially available, but CellSearch® system is the only FDA-approved for clinical use. It is an antibody-based assay, by which CTCs are isolated through a double check of positive and negative selection. A cell is identified as CTC by CellSearch if EpCAM (Epithelial Cell Adhesion Molecule)-positive, cytokeratins-positive, and CD45-negative.

For many years, CTCs count has been used alone as a prognostic tumor biomarker. Recent advantages in isolation and sequencing technologies changed this perspective, paving the way to DNA, RNA, and protein analysis at single-cell level (Heitzer et al. 2013; Lohr et al. 2014; Perakis and Speicher 2017). However, some limitations exist. CTCs' detection remains challenging, especially because of their very low concentration in blood. Both detection and enrichment steps require sensitive and specific analytic methods, made possible only with expensive technologies (Pantel and Alix-Panabières 2013; Lowes et al. 2016).

Main technologies available for ctDNA analysis are droplet digital PCR (ddPCR) and next-generation sequencing. The first is a targeted-approach, mainly used for detection of selected mutations. It is most sensitive and cost-effective, and it allows for an absolute quantification of mutant and wild-type copies. Conversely, NGS can be both targeted (gene panels) and untargeted (WES, WGS). It is complex and expensive, but it has a higher throughput that renders a more comprehensive detection of all known and unknown genomic alterations (SNVs, indels, CNAs, SVs), without preventive selection of any gene (Perakis and Speicher 2017). Very recently, the FoundationACT® assay, a 70-gene panel designed by Foundation Medicine, granted a Breakthrough Device designation by the FDA, likely to become the first liquid biopsy NGS panel to achieve regulatory approval (http://investors.foundationmedicine.com/news-releases/news-release-details/foundation-medicines-new-liquid-biopsy-assay-granted).

Like CTCs, ctDNA analysis has its disadvantages. Even if technically easier and cheaper than CTCs' count, a pre-analytical and analytical procedure validation is still lacking. A potential confounding factor is the presence of normal cell-free DNA that must be separated from cell-free tumoral DNA. Besides these technical considerations, a more relevant conceptual question about the biological meaning of ctDNA must be pointed out. Little is known about the origin of ctDNA (CTCs? Lytic, apoptotic tumor cells?). Assuming that they are released by dying tumor cells, how can they provide information about therapy-resistant clones?

In conclusion, liquid biopsy has demonstrated to be a valid surrogate of tissue sampling. Nevertheless, a scrupulous demonstration of analytic validity, clinical validity, and clinical utility is essential before its introduction in clinical practice.

5 NGS Implementation in Clinical Practice: Challenges and Limitations

The goal of each improvement in cancer knowledge is ultimately an improvement in patient's care. While the scientific value of NGS-based advancements is undoubtedly critical, clinical benefits deriving from them are still being discussed.

As previously mentioned, NGS allows us to obtain the entire sequence of cancer's exome or even genome at a reasonable price; in medical genetics, for example, WES and WGS represent an important tool to diagnose genetic and inherited disorders. But not all this information might have a role in determining the best diagnostic and therapeutic approach for cancer patients, for which smaller targeted panels are more often used in clinical practice (Jennings et al. 2017).

When designing an NGS cancer-panel, it is critical to distinguish between driver alterations and incidental, irrelevant genetic variants. This complex process, called variants' prioritization, is essentially made possible by large publicly accessible databases like COSMIC (Catalogue of Somatic Mutations in Cancer), the UCSC Cancer Genomics Browser, or the cBioPortal. These resources have been designed as a translational bridge between researchers and clinicians, to lower the barriers of access, and made comprehensible the complex data sets provided by large-scale genome projects like the TCGA or the CGP. In this field, the development of the GENIE project is certainly another step forward. This multiphase, multiyear, international project converges on a regularly updated registry containing all the existing CLIA-/ISO-certified genomic data obtained during the course of routine practice at multiple international institutions. The information provided is certainly useful for variants' prioritization, but also available for powering clinical and translational research, validating biomarkers, expanding drug labels or identifying new drug targets.

Thanks to these efforts, many NGS-based cancer panels are currently available in clinical practice. One example is the 52-gene Oncomine Focus Assay, which includes most of the genes targeted by on-market oncology drugs and published evidence. The same company offers a wider panel (161 genes), and even larger panels have been recently validated, including the FDA-approved FoundationOne CDx (F1CDx), which detects mutations in 324 genes and 2 genomic signatures in any tumor type, and the also FDA-approved MSK-IMPACT, a 468-gene assay developed by Memorial Sloan Kettering Cancer Center (MSKCC).

The best panel size for clinical practice has fueled an intense debate, since for many of the identifiable driver alterations there is still no approved drug available, and performing large panels for every cancer patient is not yet affordable. However, the improvement in cancer knowledge provided by wide mutational panels performed on a large scale might encourage such effort. Particularly helpful in this sense may be the recently published ESMO Scale for Clinical Actionability of molecular Targets (ESCAT) (Mateo et al. 2018), which proposes a classification system for molecular aberrations, dividing them between six levels of actionability and clinical usefulness, based on the strength of evidence from clinical studies. Such a scale might help prioritize some alterations, in order to design "pragmatic" and affordable panels for everyday oncology practice. Besides the size of the panel, discussion is still open regarding the clinical benefit deriving from these molecular characterizations. Large prospective studies have been conducted and are still ongoing to address this question. The SHIVA trial (Le Tourneau et al. 2015), for instance, studied the off-label use of targeted therapies in patients with any cancer type harboring matching molecular alterations; the study failed to show any benefit over standard treatments, arguing against the indiscriminate use of off-label molecules according to uncharacterized molecular alterations whose significance as driver mutations is unknown. This failure must be interpreted considering the aim of the study itself: it was not powered to evaluate if a specific drug would have any antitumor activity in a selected subgroup of patients but was only able to evaluate the efficiency of the treatment algorithm used to allocate drugs on the basis of molecular profiling. It is not a failure for precision medicine, but a demonstration of inefficacy of that treatment algorithm in improving patients' outcome.

The MOSCATO Trial (Massard et al. 2017), instead, showed an interesting benefit in terms of PFS in a subgroup of patients with hard-to-treat advanced cancers where an actionable alteration was found and a targeted therapy was available. It must be noted that the MOSCATO was a not-randomized, less-powerful trial, where patients were taken as their own controls by using the "PFS ratio" as primary endpoint. This measure is assessed by comparing the PFS reached on the targeted, experimental treatment to the PFS achieved by the most recent therapy, retrospectively assessed.

New, promising results presented during the last 2018 ASCO Congress have recently relaunched the importance of Precision Medicine in cancer care. The IMPACT (Initiative for Molecular Profiling and Advanced Cancer Therapy) trial was launched more than 10 years ago to evaluate the impact of personalized therapy in patients with hard-to-treat cancers. Among 3743 patients tested, 1307 had at least one druggable genomic alteration and received a specific matched therapy. The authors reported a median OS significantly longer in the matched-therapy group versus the nonmatched-therapy group (9.3 vs. 7.3 months), and a better median PFS (4 vs. 2.8 months). Interestingly, in the multivariate analysis the matched-targeted therapy was found to be an independent factor of longer OS, whereas mutations in the PI3K/AKT/motor pathway were an independent factor of shorter OS if compared to other alterations (NCT00851032 (Tsimberidou et al. 2018)).

A prospective validation of these results is expected by the IMPACT 2 trial, a randomized phase II study comparing the PFS achieved by patients receiving molecular-matched targeted therapy to PFS reached by patients treated with a molecular-unselected strategy (NCT02152254).

Beside this great potential, the implementation of Precision Medicine in the real-world of cancer care has several limitations. First of all, costs of NGS-based tests are still prohibitive and largely not reimbursed, representing a patient's effort as out-of-pocket expense. Costs of targeted gene panels vary widely, mainly depending on the numbers of genes sequenced. For example, a recently published nation-wide French study reported a cost ranging between €376 and €968 (Marino et al. 2018), whereas the cost-effective analysis conducted on 10 studies by Tan et al. calculated an average cost of $1609 USD per sample (range: $488–$3443 USD) (Tan et al. 2018). The authors observed that cost of sequencing is generally lower if performed in-house compared to outsourcing to a service provider.

Many concerns have been raised about the impact of these costs in terms of clinical benefit. Even if evidences for cost-effectiveness are still lacking for many cancer types, in NSCLC an upfront mutational analysis based on NGS demonstrated to be less costly and faster than a single-gene test approach. Presented at ASCO 2018, this economic model showed a saving of 2 billion dollars for US Medicare reimbursement (Pennell et al. 2018).

Accessibility to tests and drugs is another obstacle that needs to be overcome. In recent years, many national projects have been launched to facilitate test accessibility. "France Medecine Genomiques 2025" (https://www.gouvernement.fr/sites/default/files/document/document/2016/06/22.06.2016_remise_du_rapport_dyves_levy_-_france_medecine_genomique_2025.pdf) and the "100k Genomes Project from UK" (https://www.genomicsengland.co.uk/the-100000-genomes-project/) are two such examples, born to transfer resources and results of genomic medicine from clinical trials to clinical care. On the other hand, even if a patient is found to harbor a druggable mutation, the accessibility to a specific target therapy is not guaranteed outside clinical trials. Targeted agents are approved by regulatory agency more often in histology-oriented settings, being the tumor-agnostic approval of pembrolizumab is still an exception for microsatellite-unstable tumors. To solve this question, predicting biomarkers, molecular tests, and targeted drugs should be ideally developed and approved in parallel. Innovative and clever study designs have emerged with this purpose: basket, umbrella, and adaptive enrichment are state-of-the-art approaches conceived for a personalization of treatment at its best.

During the last 2018 ASCO Congress, Otis Brawley, MD and ASCO chief medical officer said: "Precision medicine has given us some things, but it has promised a lot, which it has yet to deliver." Instead of interpreting this sentence as a criticism, we want to read it as a promise. The best is yet to come.

References

Antonarakis, E. S., Lu, C., Wang, H., Luber, B., Nakazawa, M., Roeser, J. C., et al. (2014). AR-V7 and resistance to enzalutamide and abiraterone in prostate cancer. *New England Journal of Medicine, 371*(11), 1028–1038.

Atkinson, A. J., Colburn, W. A., Degruttola, V. G., Demets, D. L., Downing, G. J., Hoth, D. F., et al. (2001). Biomarkers and surrogate endpoints: Preferred definitions and conceptual framework. *Clinical Pharmacology & Therapeutics, 69*(3), 89–95.

Barata, P., Sood, A. K., & Hong, D. S. (2016). RNA-targeted therapeutics in cancer clinical trials: Current status and future directions. *Cancer Treatment Reviews, 50*, 35–47.

Barski, A., Cuddapah, S., Cui, K., Roh, T. Y., Schones, D. E., Wang, Z., et al. (2007). High-resolution profiling of histone methylations in the human genome. *Cell, 129*(4), 823–837.

Chalmers, Z. R., Connelly, C. F., Fabrizio, D., Gay, L., Ali, S. M., Ennis, R., et al. (2017). Analysis of 100,000 human cancer genomes reveals the landscape of tumor mutational burden. *Genome Medicine, 9*(1), 34.

Chandarlapaty, S., Chen, D., He, W., Sung, P., Samoila, A., You, D., et al. (2016). Prevalence of ESR1 mutations in cell-free DNA and outcomes in metastatic breast cancer: a secondary analysis of the BOLERO-2 clinical trial. *JAMA Oncology, 2*(10), 1310–1315.

Chu, D., Paoletti, C., Gersch, C., Van Den Berg, D. A., Zabransky, D. J., Cochran, R. L., et al. (2016). ESR1 mutations in circulating plasma tumor DNA from metastatic breast cancer patients. *Clinical Cancer Research, 22*(4), 993–999.

Cohen, J. D., Li, L., Wang, Y., Thoburn, C., Afsari, B., Danilova, L., et al. (2018). Detection and localization of surgically resectable cancers with a multi-analyte blood test. *Science, eaar3247.*

Cristofanilli, M., Turner, N. C., Bondarenko, I., Ro, J., Im, S. A., Masuda, N., et al. (2016). Fulvestrant plus palbociclib versus fulvestrant plus placebo for treatment of hormone-receptor-positive, HER2-negative metastatic breast cancer that progressed on previous endocrine therapy (PALOMA-3): final analysis of the multicentre, double-blind, phase 3 randomised controlled trial. *The Lancet Oncology, 17*(4), 425–439.

De Mattos-Arruda, L., Weigelt, B., Cortes, J., Won, H. H., Ng, C. K. Y., Nuciforo, P., et al. (2014). Capturing intra-tumor genetic heterogeneity by de novo mutation profiling of circulating cell-free tumor DNA: A proof-of-principle. *Annals of Oncology, 25*(9), 1729–1735.

Ding, L., Wendl, M. C., McMichael, J. F., & Raphael, B. J. (2014). Expanding the computational toolbox for mining cancer genomes. *Nature Reviews Genetics, 15*(8), 556.

Douillard, J. Y., Ostoros, G., Cobo, M., Ciuleanu, T., Cole, R., McWalter, G., et al. (2014). Gefitinib treatment in EGFR mutated caucasian NSCLC: circulating-free tumor DNA as a surrogate for determination of EGFR status. *Journal of Thoracic Oncology, 9*(9), 1345–1353.

Fehm, T., Müller, V., Aktas, B., Janni, W., Schneeweiss, A., Stickeler, E., et al. (2010). HER2 status of circulating tumor cells in patients with metastatic breast cancer: A prospective, multicenter trial. *Breast Cancer Research and Treatment, 124*(2), 403–412.

Fischer, O. M., Streit, S., Hart, S., & Ullrich, A. (2003). Beyond herceptin and gleevec. *Current Opinion in Chemical Biology, 7*(4), 490–495.

Fizazi, K., Greco, F. A., Pavlidis, N., Daugaard, G., Oien, K., & Pentheroudakis, G. (2015). Cancers of unknown primary site: ESMO Clinical Practice Guidelines for diagnosis, treatment and follow-up. *Annals of Oncology, 26*(suppl_5), v133–v138.

Fong, P. C., Boss, D. S., Yap, T. A., Tutt, A., Wu, P., Mergui-Roelvink, M., et al. (2009). Inhibition of poly (ADP-ribose) polymerase in tumors from BRCA mutation carriers. *New England Journal of Medicine, 361*(2), 123–134.

Foundation Medicine's New Liquid Biopsy Assay Granted Breakthrough Device Designation by U.S. Food and Drug Administration I Foundation Medicine, Inc. http://investors.foundationmedicine.com/news-releases/news-release-details/foundation-medicines-new-liquid-biopsy-assay-granted

FRANCE MÉDECINE GÉNOMIQUE. (2025). https://www.gouvernement.fr/sites/default/files/document/document/2016/06/22.06.2016_remise_du_rapport_dyves_levy_-_france_medecine_genomique_2025.pdf

Fribbens, C., O'Leary, B., Kilburn, L., Hrebien, S., Garcia-Murillas, I., Beaney, M., … & Jiang, J. (2016). Plasma ESR1 mutations and the treatment of estrogen receptor-positive advanced breast cancer.

Gandara, D. R., Kowanetz, M., Mok, T. S. K., Rittmeyer, A., Fehrenbacher, L., Fabrizio, D., et al. (2017). 1295OBlood-based biomarkers for cancer immunotherapy: Tumor mutational burden in blood (bTMB) is associated with improved atezolizumab (atezo) efficacy in 2L+ NSCLC (POPLAR and OAK). *Annals of Oncology, 28*(suppl_5).

Garcia-Murillas, I., Schiavon, G., Weigelt, B., Ng, C., Hrebien, S., Cutts, R. J., et al. (2015). Mutation tracking in circulating tumor DNA predicts relapse in early breast cancer. *Science Translational Medicine, 7*(302), 302ra133-302ra133.

Gillessen, S., Attard, G., Beer, T. M., Beltran, H., Bossi, A., Bristow, R., et al. (2018). Management of patients with advanced prostate cancer: The report of the Advanced Prostate Cancer Consensus Conference APCCC 2017. *European Urology, 73*(2), 178–211.

Gomes, A. Q., Nolasco, S., & Soares, H. (2013). Non-coding RNAs: Multi-tasking molecules in the cell. *International Journal of Molecular Sciences, 14*(8), 16010–16039.

Gonzalez-Perez, A., Mustonen, V., Reva, B., Ritchie, G. R., Creixell, P., Karchin, R., et al. (2013). Computational approaches to identify functional genetic variants in cancer genomes. *Nature Methods, 10*(8), 723.

Green, E. D., Watson, J. D., & Collins, F. S. (2015). Human Genome Project: Twenty-five years of big biology. *Nature News, 526*(7571), 29.

Greenman, C., Stephens, P., Smith, R., Dalgliesh, G. L., Hunter, C., Bignell, G., et al. (2007). Patterns of somatic mutation in human cancer genomes. *Nature, 446*(7132), 153.

Gröbe, A., Blessmann, M., Hanken, H., Friedrich, R. E., Schön, G., Wikner, J., et al. (2014). Prognostic relevance of circulating tumor cells in blood and disseminated tumor cells in bone marrow of patients with squamous cell carcinoma of the oral cavity. *Clinical Cancer Research, 20*(2), 425–433.

Hainsworth, J. D., Rubin, M. S., Spigel, D. R., Boccia, R. V., Raby, S., Quinn, R., & Greco, F. A. (2012). Molecular gene expression profiling to predict the tissue of origin and direct site-specific therapy in patients with carcinoma of unknown primary site: a prospective trial of the Sarah Cannon research institute. *Journal of Clinical Oncology, 31*(2), 217–223.

Hamilton, E. P., Patel, M. R., Armstrong, A. C., Baird, R. D., Jhaveri, K., Hoch, M., et al. (2018). A first in human study of the new oral selective estrogen receptor degrader AZD9496 for HR+/HER2− advanced breast cancer. *Clinical Cancer Research, clincanres-3102*.

Heitzer, E., Auer, M., Gasch, C., Pichler, M., Ulz, P., Hoffmann, E. M., et al. (2013). Complex tumor genomes inferred from single circulating tumor cells by array-CGH and next-generation sequencing. *Cancer Research*.

Hellmann, M. D., Callahan, M. K., Awad, M. M., Calvo, E., Ascierto, P. A., Atmaca, A., et al. (2018a). Tumor mutational burden and efficacy of nivolumab monotherapy and in combination with ipilimumab in small-cell lung cancer. *Cancer Cell, 33*(5), 853–861.

Hellmann, M. D., Ciuleanu, T. E., Pluzanski, A., Lee, J. S., Otterson, G. A., Audigier-Valette, C., et al. (2018b). Nivolumab plus ipilimumab in lung cancer with a high tumor mutational burden. *New England Journal of Medicine*.

Hustedt, N., & Durocher, D. (2017). The control of DNA repair by the cell cycle. *Nature Cell Biology, 19*(1), 1.

Ignatiadis, M., & Dawson, S. J. (2014). Circulating tumor cells and circulating tumor DNA for precision medicine: Dream or reality? *Annals of Oncology, 25*(12), 2304–2313.

Jasin, M., & Rothstein, R. (2013). Repair of strand breaks by homologous recombination. *Cold Spring Harbor Perspectives in Biology, a012740*.

Jennings, L. J., Arcila, M. E., Corless, C., Kamel-Reid, S., Lubin, I. M., Pfeifer, J., et al. (2017). Guidelines for validation of next-generation sequencing–based oncology panels: A joint consensus recommendation of the Association for Molecular Pathology and College of American Pathologists. *The Journal of Molecular Diagnostics, 19*(3), 341–365.

Jeselsohn, R., Yelensky, R., Buchwalter, G., Frampton, G., Meric-Bernstam, F., Gonzalez-Angulo, A. M., et al. (2014). Emergence of constitutively active estrogen receptor-α mutations in pretreated advanced estrogen receptor–positive breast cancer. *Clinical Cancer Research, 20*(7), 1757–1767.

Johnson, D. B., Frampton, G. M., Rioth, M. J., Yusko, E., Xu, Y., Guo, X., et al. (2016). Targeted next generation sequencing identifies markers of response to PD-1 blockade. *Cancer Immunology Research*.

Johnson, J. R., Bross, P., Cohen, M., Rothmann, M., Chen, G., Zajicek, A., et al. (2003). Approval summary: Imatinib mesylate capsules for treatment of adult patients with newly diagnosed Philadelphia chromosome-positive chronic myelogenous leukemia in chronic phase. *Clinical Cancer Research, 9*(6), 1972–1979.

Johnston, S. R., Kilburn, L. S., Ellis, P., Dodwell, D., Cameron, D., Hayward, L., et al. (2013). Fulvestrant plus anastrozole or placebo versus exemestane alone after progression on non-steroidal aromatase inhibitors in postmenopausal patients with hormone-receptor-positive locally advanced or metastatic breast cancer (SoFEA): a composite, multicentre, phase 3 randomised trial. *The Lancet Oncology, 14*(10), 989–998.

Kinzler, K. W., & Vogelstein, B. (1996). Lessons from hereditary colorectal cancer. *Cell, 87*(2), 159–170.

Koboldt, D. C., Fulton, R. S., McLellan, M. D., Schmidt, H., Kalicki-Veizer, J., McMichael, J. F., et al. (2012). Comprehensive molecular portraits of human breast tumours. *Nature, 490*(7418), 61–70.

Kuang, Y., Rogers, A., Yeap, B. Y., Wang, L., Makrigiorgos, M., Vetrand, K., et al. (2009). Noninvasive detection of EGFR T790M in gefitinib or erlotinib resistant non–small cell lung cancer. *Clinical Cancer Research, 15*(8), 2630–2636.

Landau, D. A., Carter, S. L., Stojanov, P., McKenna, A., Stevenson, K., Lawrence, M. S., et al. (2013). Evolution and impact of subclonal mutations in chronic lymphocytic leukemia. *Cell, 152*(4), 714–726.

Le, D. T., Durham, J. N., Smith, K. N., Wang, H., Bartlett, B. R., Aulakh, L. K., et al. (2017). Mismatch repair deficiency predicts response of solid tumors to PD-1 blockade. *Science, 357*(6349), 409–413.

Le Tourneau, C., Delord, J. P., Gonçalves, A., Gavoille, C., Dubot, C., Isambert, N., et al. (2015). Molecularly targeted therapy based on tumour molecular profiling versus conventional therapy for advanced cancer (SHIVA): A multicentre, open-label, proof-of-concept, randomised, controlled phase 2 trial. *The Lancet Oncology, 16*(13), 1324–1334.

Lebofsky, R., Decraene, C., Bernard, V., Kamal, M., Blin, A., Leroy, Q., et al. (2015). Circulating tumor DNA as a non-invasive substitute to metastasis biopsy for tumor genotyping and personalized medicine in a prospective trial across all tumor types. *Molecular Oncology, 9*(4), 783–790.

Lister, R., O'Malley, R. C., Tonti-Filippini, J., Gregory, B. D., Berry, C. C., Millar, A. H., & Ecker, J. R. (2008). Highly integrated single-base resolution maps of the epigenome in Arabidopsis. *Cell, 133*(3), 523–536.

Lohr, J. G., Adalsteinsson, V. A., Cibulskis, K., Choudhury, A. D., Rosenberg, M., Cruz-Gordillo, P., et al. (2014). Whole-exome sequencing of circulating tumor cells provides a window into metastatic prostate cancer. *Nature Biotechnology, 32*(5), 479.

Lowes, L. E., Bratman, S. V., Dittamore, R., Done, S., Kelley, S. O., Mai, S., et al. (2016). Circulating tumor cells (CTC) and cell-free DNA (cfDNA) workshop 2016: Scientific opportunities and logistics for cancer clinical trial incorporation. *International Journal of Molecular Sciences, 17*(9), 1505.

Lynch, H. T., Smyrk, T. C., Watson, P., Lanspa, S. J., Lynch, J. F., Lynch, P. M., et al. (1993). Genetics, natural history, tumor spectrum, and pathology of hereditary nonpolyposis colorectal cancer: an updated review. *Gastroenterology, 104*(5), 1535–1549.

Margulies, M., Egholm, M., Altman, W. E., Attiya, S., Bader, J. S., Bemben, L. A., et al. (2005). Genome sequencing in microfabricated high-density picolitre reactors. *Nature, 437*(7057), 376.

Marino, P., Touzani, R., Perrier, L., Rouleau, E., Kossi, D. S., Zhaomin, Z., et al. (2018). Cost of cancer diagnosis using next-generation sequencing targeted gene panels in routine practice: a nationwide French study. *European Journal of Human Genetics, 26*(3), 314.

Mariotto, A. B., Etzioni, R., Hurlbert, M., Penberthy, L., & Mayer, M. (2017). Estimation of the number of women living with metastatic breast cancer in the United States. *Cancer Epidemiology and Prevention Biomarkers*.

Markowski, M. C., Silberstein, J. L., Eshleman, J. R., Eisenberger, M. A., Luo, J., & Antonarakis, E. S. (2017). Clinical utility of CLIA-grade AR-V7 testing in patients with metastatic castration-resistant prostate cancer. *JCO Precision Oncology, 1*, 1–9.

Massard, C., Loriot, Y., & Fizazi, K. (2011). Carcinomas of an unknown primary origin—Diagnosis and treatment. *Nature Reviews Clinical Oncology, 8*(12), 701.

Massard, C., Michiels, S., Ferté, C., Le Deley, M. C., Lacroix, L., Hollebecque, A., et al. (2017). High-throughput genomics and clinical outcome in hard-to-treat advanced cancers: Results of the MOSCATO 01 trial. *Cancer Discovery*.

Mastoraki, S., Strati, A., Tzanikou, E., Chimonidou, M., Politaki, E., Voutsina, A., et al. (2018). ESR1 methylation: A liquid biopsy–based epigenetic assay for the follow-up of patients with metastatic breast cancer receiving endocrine treatment. *Clinical Cancer Research, 24*(6), 1500–1510.

Mateo, J., Chakravarty, D., Dienstmann, R., Jezdic, S., Gonzalez-Perez, A., Lopez-Bigas, N., et al. (2018). A framework to rank genomic alterations as targets for cancer precision medicine: the ESMO Scale for Clinical Actionability of molecular Targets (ESCAT). *Annals of Oncology, 29*(9), 1895–1902.

Merenbakh-Lamin, K., Ben-Baruch, N., Yeheskel, A., Dvir, A., Soussan-Gutman, L., Jeselsohn, R., et al. (2013). D538G mutation in estrogen receptor-α: A novel mechanism for acquired endocrine resistance in breast cancer. *Cancer Research*.

Misale, S., Yaeger, R., Hobor, S., Scala, E., Janakiraman, M., Liska, D., et al. (2012). Emergence of KRAS mutations and acquired resistance to anti-EGFR therapy in colorectal cancer. *Nature, 486*(7404), 532.

Mok, T. S., Wu, Y. L., Ahn, M. J., Garassino, M. C., Kim, H. R., Ramalingam, S. S., et al. (2017). Osimertinib or platinum–pemetrexed in EGFR T790M–positive lung cancer. *New England Journal of Medicine, 376*(7), 629–640.

Mouliere, F., El Messaoudi, S., Gongora, C., Guedj, A. S., Robert, B., Del Rio, M., et al. (2013). Circulating cell-free DNA from colorectal cancer patients may reveal high KRAS or BRAF mutation load. *Translational Oncology, 6*(3), 319–328.

Moynahan, M. E., Chiu, J. W., Koller, B. H., & Jasin, M. (1999). Brca1 controls homology-directed DNA repair. *Molecular Cell, 4*(4), 511–518.

Moynahan, M. E., Pierce, A. J., & Jasin, M. (2001). BRCA2 is required for homology-directed repair of chromosomal breaks. *Molecular Cell, 7*(2), 263–272.

Nakamura, T., Sueoka-Aragane, N., Iwanaga, K., Sato, A., Komiya, K., Kobayashi, N., et al. (2012). Application of a highly sensitive detection system for epidermal growth factor receptor mutations in plasma DNA. *Journal of Thoracic Oncology, 7*(9), 1369–1381.

Nastaly, P., Ruf, C. G., Becker, P., Bednarz-Knoll, N., Stoupiec, M., Kavsur, R., et al. (2014). Circulating tumor cells in patients with testicular germ cell tumors. *Clinical Cancer Research*, clincanres-2819.

National Comprehensive Cancer Network. Non-small cell lung cancer (Version 6.2018). https://www.nccn.org/professionals/physician_gls/pdf/nscl.pdf

Nowell, P. C. (1976). The clonal evolution of tumor cell populations. *Science, 194*(4260), 23–28.

O'Kane, G. M., Connor, A. A., & Gallinger, S. (2017). Characterization, detection, and treatment approaches for homologous recombination deficiency in cancer. *Trends in Molecular Medicine*.

Olsson, E., Winter, C., George, A., Chen, Y., Howlin, J., Tang, M. H. E., et al. (2015). Serial monitoring of circulating tumor DNA in patients with primary breast cancer for detection of occult metastatic disease. *EMBO Molecular Medicine, 7*(8), 1034–1047.

Oxnard, G. R., Paweletz, C. P., Kuang, Y., Mach, S. L., O'Connell, A., Messineo, M. M., et al. (2014). Noninvasive detection of response and resistance in EGFR-mutant lung cancer using quantitative next-generation genotyping of cell-free plasma DNA. *Clinical Cancer Research*.

Pantel, K., & Alix-Panabières, C. (2013). Real-time liquid biopsy in cancer patients: Fact or fiction? *Cancer Research*.

Paoletti, C., Muniz, M. C., Thomas, D. G., Griffith, K. A., Kidwell, K. M., Tokudome, N., et al. (2015). Development of circulating tumor cell-endocrine therapy index in patients with hormone receptor–positive breast cancer. *Clinical Cancer Research, 21*(11), 2487–2498.

Pennell, N. A., Mutebi, A., Zhou, Z. Y., Ricculli, M. L., Tang, W., Wang, H., … & Otterson, G. A. (2018). Economic impact of next generation sequencing vs sequential single-gene testing modalities to detect genomic alterations in metastatic non-small cell lung cancer using a decision analytic model.

Perakis, S., & Speicher, M. R. (2017). Emerging concepts in liquid biopsies. *BMC Medicine, 15*(1), 75.

Rack, B., Schindlbeck, C., Jückstock, J., Andergassen, U., Hepp, P., Zwingers, T., et al. (2014). Circulating tumor cells predict survival in early average-to-high risk breast cancer patients. *JNCI: Journal of the National Cancer Institute, 106*(5).

Raphael, B. J., Dobson, J. R., Oesper, L., & Vandin, F. (2014). Identifying driver mutations in sequenced cancer genomes: Computational approaches to enable precision medicine. *Genome Medicine, 6*(1), 5.

Reck, M., Hagiwara, K., Han, B., Tjulandin, S., Grohé, C., Yokoi, T., et al. (2016). ctDNA determination of EGFR mutation status in European and Japanese patients with advanced NSCLC: The ASSESS study. *Journal of Thoracic Oncology, 11*(10), 1682–1689.

Reinert, T., Schøler, L. V., Thomsen, R., Tobiasen, H., Vang, S., Nordentoft, I., et al. (2016). Analysis of circulating tumour DNA to monitor disease burden following colorectal cancer surgery. *Gut, 65*(4), 625–634.

Rink, M., Chun, F. K., Dahlem, R., Soave, A., Minner, S., Hansen, J., et al. (2012). Prognostic role and HER2 expression of circulating tumor cells in peripheral blood of patients prior to radical cystectomy: A prospective study. *European Urology, 61*(4), 810–817.

Rizvi, N. A., Hellmann, M. D., Snyder, A., Kvistborg, P., Makarov, V., Havel, J. J., et al. (2015). Mutational landscape determines sensitivity to PD-1 blockade in non–small cell lung cancer. *Science, 348*(6230), 124–128.

Robinson, D. R., Wu, Y. M., Vats, P., Su, F., Lonigro, R. J., Cao, X., et al. (2013). Activating ESR1 mutations in hormone-resistant metastatic breast cancer. *Nature Genetics, 45*(12), 1446.

Robson, M., Im, S. A., Senkus, E., Xu, B., Domchek, S. M., Masuda, N., et al. (2017). Olaparib for metastatic breast cancer in patients with a germline BRCA mutation. *New England Journal of Medicine, 377*(6), 523–533.

Rosenberg, J. E., Hoffman-Censits, J., Powles, T., Van Der Heijden, M. S., Balar, A. V., Necchi, A., et al. (2016). Atezolizumab in patients with locally advanced and metastatic urothelial carcinoma who have progressed following treatment with platinum-based chemotherapy: a single-arm, multicentre, phase 2 trial. *The Lancet, 387*(10031), 1909–1920.

Sanger, F., Nicklen, S., & Coulson, A. R. (1977). DNA sequencing with chain-terminating inhibitors. *Proceedings of the national academy of sciences, 74*(12), 5463–5467.

Scher, H. I., Lu, D., Schreiber, N. A., Louw, J., Graf, R. P., Vargas, H. A., et al. (2016). Association of AR-V7 on circulating tumor cells as a treatment-specific biomarker with outcomes and survival in castration-resistant prostate cancer. *JAMA Oncology, 2*(11), 1441–1449.

Schiavon, G., Hrebien, S., Garcia-Murillas, I., Cutts, R. J., Pearson, A., Tarazona, N., et al. (2015). Analysis of ESR1 mutation in circulating tumor DNA demonstrates evolution during therapy for metastatic breast cancer. *Science Translational Medicine, 7*(313), 313ra182-313ra182.

Schulze, K., Gasch, C., Staufer, K., Nashan, B., Lohse, A. W., Pantel, K., et al. (2013). Presence of EpCAM-positive circulating tumor cells as biomarker for systemic disease strongly correlates to survival in patients with hepatocellular carcinoma. *International Journal of Cancer, 133*(9), 2165–2171.

Shin, S. H., Bode, A. M., & Dong, Z. (2017). Precision medicine: the foundation of future cancer therapeutics. *NPJ Precision Oncology, 1*(1), 12.

Siravegna, G., Mussolin, B., Buscarino, M., Corti, G., Cassingena, A., Crisafulli, G., et al. (2015). Clonal evolution and resistance to EGFR blockade in the blood of colorectal cancer patients. *Nature Medicine, 21*(7), 795.

Snyder, A., Makarov, V., Merghoub, T., Yuan, J., Zaretsky, J. M., Desrichard, A., et al. (2014). Genetic basis for clinical response to CTLA-4 blockade in melanoma. *New England Journal of Medicine, 371*(23), 2189–2199.

Swanton, C., Soria, J. C., Bardelli, A., Biankin, A., Caldas, C., Chandarlapaty, S., et al. (2016). Consensus on precision medicine for metastatic cancers: a report from the MAP conference. *Annals of Oncology, 27*(8), 1443–1448.

Swisher, E. M., Lin, K. K., Oza, A. M., Scott, C. L., Giordano, H., Sun, J., et al. (2017). Rucaparib in relapsed, platinum-sensitive high-grade ovarian carcinoma (ARIEL2 Part 1): an international, multicentre, open-label, phase 2 trial. *The Lancet Oncology, 18*(1), 75–87.

Szostak, J. W., Orr-Weaver, T. L., Rothstein, R. J., & Stahl, F. W. (1983). The double-strand-break repair model for recombination. *Cell, 33*(1), 25–35.

Tan, O., Shrestha, R., Cunich, M., & Schofield, D. J. (2018). Application of next-generation sequencing to improve cancer management: A review of the clinical effectiveness and cost-effectiveness. *Clinical Genetics, 93*(3), 533–544.

Taniguchi, K., Uchida, J., Nishino, K., Kumagai, T., Okuyama, T., Okami, J., et al. (2011). Quantitative detection of EGFR mutations in circulating tumor DNA derived from lung adenocarcinomas. *Clinical Cancer Research.*

The 100,000 Genomes Project | Genomics England. https://www.genomicsengland.co.uk/the-100000-genomes-project/

Thibodeau, S. N., Bren, G., & Schaid, D. (1993). Microsatellite instability in cancer of the proximal colon. *Science, 260*(5109), 816–819.

TracerX | Tracking Cancer Evolution through study. http://tracerx.co.uk/

Tsimberidou, A. M., Hong, D. S., Wheler, J. J., Falchook, G. S., Naing, A., Fu, S., … & Nogueras-Gonzalez, G. M. (2018). Precision medicine: Clinical outcomes including long-term survival according to the pathway targeted and treatment period–The IMPACT study.

Turner, N. C., Jiang, Y., O'Leary, B., Hrebien, S., Cristofanilli, M., Andre, F., … & Bartlett, C. H. (2016). Efficacy of palbociclib plus fulvestrant (P+ F) in patients (pts) with metastatic breast cancer (MBC) and ESR1 mutations (mus) in circulating tumor DNA (ctDNA).

Vanderwalde, A., Spetzler, D., Xiao, N., Gatalica, Z., & Marshall, J. (2018). Microsatellite instability status determined by next-generation sequencing and compared with PD-L1 and tumor mutational burden in 11,348 patients. *Cancer Medicine, 7*(3), 746–756.

Varghese, A. M., Arora, A., Capanu, M., Camacho, N., Won, H. H., Zehir, A., et al. (2017). Clinical and molecular characterization of patients with cancer of unknown primary in the modern era. *Annals of Oncology, 28*(12), 3015–3021.

Velcheti, V., Kim, E. S., Mekhail, T., Dakhil, C., Stella, P. J., Shen, X., … & Phan, S. C. (2018). Prospective clinical evaluation of blood-based tumor mutational burden (bTMB) as a predictive biomarker for atezolizumab (atezo) in 1L non-small cell lung cancer (NSCLC): Interim B-F1RST results.

Vilar, E., & Gruber, S. B. (2010). Microsatellite instability in colorectal cancer—the stable evidence. *Nature Reviews Clinical Oncology, 7*(3), 153.

Vogelstein, B., Papadopoulos, N., Velculescu, V. E., Zhou, S., Diaz, L. A., & Kinzler, K. W. (2013). Cancer genome landscapes. *Science, 339*(6127), 1546–1558.

Wang, Z., Gerstein, M., & Snyder, M. (2009). RNA-Seq: a revolutionary tool for transcriptomics. *Nature Reviews Genetics, 10*(1), 57.

Weis, K. E., Ekena, K., Thomas, J. A., Lazennec, G., & Katzenellenbogen, B. S. (1996). Constitutively active human estrogen receptors containing amino acid substitutions for tyrosine 537 in the receptor protein. *Molecular Endocrinology, 10*(11), 1388–1398.

Morris, J. R. (2001). Genes, genetics, and epigenetics: a correspondence. *Science, 293*(5532), 1103–1105.

Yang, M., Forbes, M. E., Bitting, R. L., O'neill, S. S., Chou, P. C., Topaloglu, U., et al. (2017). Incorporating blood-based liquid biopsy information into cancer staging: time for a TNMB system? *Annals of Oncology, 29*(2), 311–323.

Yap, T. A., Gerlinger, M., Futreal, P. A., Pusztai, L., & Swanton, C. (2012). Intratumor heterogeneity: seeing the wood for the trees. *Science Translational Medicine, 4*(127), 127ps10-127ps10.

Yokobori, T., Iinuma, H., Shimamura, T., Imoto, S., Sugimachi, K., Ishii, H., et al. (2013). Plastin3 is a novel marker for circulating tumor cells undergoing the epithelial-mesenchymal transition and is associated with colorectal cancer prognosis. *Cancer Research*, canres-0326.

Chapter 9
User-Centered Design Approaches and Methods for P5 eHealth

Stefano Triberti and Eleonora Brivio

1 Introduction

As seen throughout this book, the P5 approach to healthcare technology calls for devices that are preventive, predictive, personalized, participatory, and sensitive to psycho-cognitive aspects of both interaction with technology itself and health issues (Gorini and Pravettoni 2011; Pravettoni and Gorini 2011). The previous contributions have deepened these concepts through historical, theoretical, and methodological information: for example, it has been said that innovative devices (e.g., wearable technology, and/or Ambient Intelligence applications) may help to detect and analyze not only the progress of disease, but also patients' state in terms of emotional activation, observable behavior, and subjectively reported preferences. Moreover, previous contributions explained how technological devices can be based on personal characteristics, both in their interactive physical properties (i.e., to promote effective ergonomics) and in the content of digital stimuli (Vergani et al. 2019).

In general, it has been said that eHealth tools should be *tailored* on patients' characteristics in order to be deeply effective and obtain desirable results in an acceptable amount of time (cf. Chap. 1). Such a message could be difficult to understand or to translate into practice for those stakeholders who are interested in the development of eHealth tools, but who are not expert in the design of technology. The idea of "tailoring technology on users" may just look like a "way of saying" with no actual impact (or no practical one) on health technology development and

S. Triberti (✉)
Department of Oncology and Hemato-Oncology, University of Milan, Milan, Italy

Applied Research Division for Cognitive and Psychological Science,
European Institute of Oncology (IEO) IRCCS, Milan, Italy
e-mail: stefano.triberti@unimi.it

E. Brivio
Department of Psychology, Università Cattolica del Sacro Cuore, Milan, Italy

G. Pravettoni, S. Triberti (eds.), *P5 eHealth: An Agenda for the Health Technologies of the Future*, https://doi.org/10.1007/978-3-030-27994-3_9

implementation. What does it actually mean to tailor technology on its users? There are at least four possible answers readers could have considered while reading this book and considering the P5 approach to eHealth:

1. Technology developers should keep in mind the fundamental characteristics of the diagnosis and of its consequences on everyday life (both physical and psychological), in order to design tools that could be used effectively and causing no harm.
2. The eHealth tools of the future should include personalization features and pleasant/engaging aspects so the users could develop a positive attitude toward use and possibly be driven toward a higher rate of acceptance and adoption in the long term (cf. Chap. 4).
3. The eHealth tools of the future should be developed with features allowing modifications at later stages of interventions, according to users' feedback.
4. Technology developers should keep themselves up-to-date with scientific literature on development and effectiveness of eHealth solutions, in order to address issues that are known within the literature, especially for what regards factors that may promote or hinder acceptance and adoption among users.

All these possible answers feature directions that are very important and certainly deserve eHealth developers' and stakeholders' consideration; however, none of them could be considered sufficient from the point of view expressed by the P5 eHealth approach and its indications for technology design.

Specifically, the first response has merit because it considers the medical characteristics of chronic diseases and the fact that they could have important influences on everyday life, both physical and psychological; however, it is not only the pathology that influences effective human–technology interaction, neither acceptance nor adoption in the long term; patients are not "only patients"; despite an eHealth tool/technology could be designed in order to be used by patients' whose lifestyle is influenced by the onset and continuous presence of a chronic disease, also personal preferences, habits and behaviors could get in the way of effective usage, or the technology could be inadequate to contextual factors that have nothing to do with users' health status. Moreover, at an organizational level, it is not possible to expect that technology designers would develop health professionals' specific knowledge and competences, and neither that health professionals would be fully employed in the design and development of technology.

The second response values psychological aspects of interaction more, but fails in giving specific guidelines to include these in the design/development process; moreover, it seems to not consider that psychological aspects such as preferences and positive emotions are transient and could change over the course of time, possibly making eHealth solutions no more adequate to users in the long term.

The third response takes some steps further by acknowledging the *iterative* nature that an evolved conception of technology design often features: certainly, eHealth design should take into consideration that modifications could be necessary at every step of implementation and interaction, so that the design process does not end with the final prototype. However, this response does not provide specifications on which kind of information one should consider for modifying or redesigning technology; is "users' feedback" sufficient? The next pages will show that the response to this last question could not be so simple.

Finally, the fourth answer points out one very important aspect, that is, eHealth development should be based on scientific information, not only on the designers' skills and creativity; however, it is important to appreciate that not even scientific literature is sufficient to inform design; indeed, scientific results are necessarily based on samples that tend to oversee individual characteristics and differences. Of course, eHealth development needs to be based on general guidelines but, in order to be very effective and to augment its possibilities to be adopted, it should be able to consider specific cases and fine-grained practice information that often could be not included in scientific reports.

In conclusion, "tailoring technologies on users" is a guiding concept that possibly includes all the considerations outlined above, but should go beyond these including specific guidelines for practice. Therefore, this chapter is aimed at outlining methodological consideration to translate such concept into practice, and to give specific information on how this "tailoring" could be enacted in the eHealth project, from the very first steps of design to final implementation. More specifically, the proposal of this chapter relies on the methods of so-called User-Centered Design.

2 From Ergonomics to User-Centered Design

In our opinion, the best way to introduce the concept of User-Centered Design is to locate it in the history of technology evaluation. Indeed, technologies (especially those designed to be used in the healthcare context) always need to be evaluated, which means, it should be demonstrated whether they are able to (help human users to) achieve their aims, or not.

Historically, the so-called Scientific Study of Work emerged during the Industrial Revolution, which can be considered the first organized way to evaluate technologies (Nickerson 1999; Triberti and Brivio 2017): its aims were to analyze human work (often mediated by industrial technologies) in order to divide it in simple actions that could be taught to the workers in order to improve productivity.

Subsequently, ergonomics (mostly in Europe) and Human Factors (mostly in the United States) emerged in 1900, as disciplines devoted to improve physical/anatomical and cognitive aspects of technology-mediated work in order to improve product quality and productivity but also safety and possibly subjective satisfaction (Karwowski 2012; Sharit 2006; Wilson 2000).

In the 1980s, Usability arose as a "simplified" form of ergonomics focused on Industrial Design, namely, as a discipline interested in empowering the interface of common-use objects, products and services so to make it easy to use and immediately comprehensible for customers, stakeholders, and users (Triberti and Brivio 2017): usability experts such as Jakob Nielsen and Donald Norman set the basis for the evaluation of the "things" and tools all of us use every day, and generated the idea that easiness of use is more important for artifacts than other properties such as originality and aesthetic beauty (Nielsen 1999, 2003; Norman 2002).

However, more recent development of the disciplines and methods associated to tools and technologies highlighted that easiness-of-use is not the sole criterion to be taken into consideration when evaluating technology: *User Experience* (UX) is the umbrella term used nowadays to identify methodological approaches that recognize the role of additional factors such as emotion/affection/pleasure (e.g., people can use nonusable objects if they "love" them) and context (e.g., besides usability of interfaces, tools can be more or less adequate to physical, social, or cultural features of situations of use) (Benyon et al. 2005; Hassenzahl 2008; Lee et al. 2008; Triberti and Brivio 2017).

This development led to the global recognition that evaluation of technology should not take into account "functioning" only, but a multiplicity of criteria to quantify effectiveness: these are at least quality, safety, easiness-of-use, emotions (positive, or if necessarily negative, possible to manage for users), adequacy to context (physical, social, cultural), accessibility (e.g., technology could be used by various populations, people with disability included).

Obviously, evaluating all of these characteristics in technology, taking into account that partial or total redesign could be called for when one or more of the criteria appear insufficient, could be very costly in terms of time and resources (Herstatt and Von Hippel 1992; Pavelin et al. 2012); however, designers, developers, and stakeholders could consider important criteria for technology effectiveness *in advance*, which means, the design itself could be based on user research data, so not only on preexistent ideas (about users, contexts, related activities, and the issue to be addressed by technology) or the creativity and intelligence of the designers. Exactly this concept is at the core of *User-Centered Design* (UCD henceforth) (Garrett 2010; Lowdermilk 2013; Triberti and Brivio 2017; Triberti and Liberati 2014), a broad term that encompasses any design project in which users and users research influence how the design itself takes place. According to Garrett (2010), UCD could be depicted as a strategy that (in a "perfect" scenario) allows for any possible issue or variable to not escape the designer's awareness. In other words, implementing UCD means that users should be involved from the very steps of design in order to provide valuable information for the design itself, not just in the last steps of implementation to evaluate some already-developed prototype (Abras et al. 2004). Although the term UCD is relatively old (Norman and Draper used it for the first time in the 1980s already) (Norman and Draper 1986), it developed into a discipline in more recent times, consistently with the semi-standardization of methods and tools devoted to analyze users' needs before design.

The next section would be devoted to introduce some typical UCD tools/techniques that could be adapted to serve eHealth design and development: taking into account the importance of the other aspects highlighted by the answers above (i.e., attention to literature, consideration of disease/illness-related issues, user engagement, iterative prototyping), the application of such techniques could help eHealth developers to tailor technologies on their users, in order to assure not only positive functioning, but also the implementation of the P5 as described in this book.

2.1 Interaction Factors

As Hesse and Shneiderman say (Hesse and Shneiderman 2007), during the pioneering days of eHealth, the question was often about what the *computer* could do; eHealth pioneers posed technical questions about computers, the Internet, and software's capability to help patients keep trace of their own medications/therapy and of their disease. During the next phase, crucial questions concern what *people* can do (and, we would add, what they cannot).

This concept is true in many senses, but in this section we focus on interaction aspects only. As previously said, the history of technology evaluation featured *Usability* as a discipline interested in developing interfaces that are easy to understand and to use for the final users. Certainly, usability is a very important characteristic that is currently taken into consideration when evaluating the adequacy and effectiveness of eHealth solutions: a number of studies have been published focusing on methods and results about medical informatics usability (Gerdes et al. 2014; Goldberg et al. 2011; Vorderstrasse et al. 2016). However, many studies just employ usability questionnaires with final users when the technology is already designed (as a prototype, or even as a final version) and it is often not clear whether these data will influence actual modification or redesign of the evaluated platforms.

Usability questionnaires (such as, e.g., the SUS (Brooke 1996)) certainly are useful tools to get, as the author says, a "quick and dirty" index about the easiness-of-use of some system or application; nevertheless, they are not conceived to give a "full" usability evaluation. Let us say, for example, one obtains a average-to-high value of usability basing on participants filling in a given questionnaire: what does this mean? This is only a general evaluation participants performed by responding to general questions, but no information has been provided about specific, more or less serious, more or less frequent system usage issues. Indeed, typical questions of such usability questionnaires are: "Were you able to use the system without effort?" or "State on a scale from 1 to 10 how much you felt to be able to obtain the system goal by using the system"; obviously, responses to such questions refer to a general evaluation but do not account for specific issues that could prevent users to achieve their own objectives in real-life contexts.

For this reason, the correct way to examine usability is to implement specific research methods, which typically are divided into two categories, namely, usability *inspection* and *testing* methods.

Usability inspection refers to those methods performed by evaluators, without the involvement of final users; these are constituted by guidelines and rules to analyze interfaces systematically, in order to account for usability problems that may escape a general, nonspecialized exploration. Currently, the main usability inspection methods still used are the *cognitive walkthrough* (which is based on exploring each function of the interface in sequence, reporting any possible problems encountered by a hypothetical user) and *heuristics analysis* (which is a global, holistic analysis of interface).

Cognitive walkthrough (Kushniruk et al. 2015) entails a checklist to be followed by evaluators who put themselves in the shoes of users, accounting for each possible action that the user would take with the interface and signaling any possible mistake or interaction issue. Differently, heuristic evaluation is based on a list of general criteria interfaces should respect in order to guarantee effective usage. A number of heuristics lists are available, such as the generic (and probably most used) by Nielsen (1995) and others for specific technologies or domains (Hermawati and Lawson 2016).

Another option (that could be also used in conjunction with inspection methods) is *usability testing*, which constitutes any technique for evaluation that involves final users who interact with the interface in systematic and more or less controlled contexts, in order to identify usability issues by a critical evaluation of actual interaction; usability testing could employ a number of methods and tools for registering usability issues, ranging from physiological signals to interviewing the participants to observation of behavior (e.g., counting the number of errors) (Smilowitz et al. 1994).

With regard to the evaluation of interaction factors, the main suggestion coming from the P5 approach is not to "resolve" such issues by basic evaluations such as using a usability questionnaire alone; on the contrary, evaluators should be activated in any phase of the development process. Specifically, usability inspection and testing methods can be applied at different phases of conceptualization of the interface and prototyping, in order to modify interaction issue *in itinere*.

2.2 *Motivation and Emotion*

User experience is not limited to usability. As explained in the sections above, User Experience (as a discipline) emerged when the role of additional factors was explicitly recognized. Indeed, it is not enough for an interface to be easy to use, especially if what is expected is to promote long-term usage. If one would plan to use technologies to change patients' everyday life, in order to positively influence their own lifestyle and care process, then eHealth resources should be also engaging, pleasant, or even self-actualizing.

According to the Positive Technology paradigm (Riva et al. 2016), technologies can be used to structure, augment, or replace users' experience with digital resources, in order to improve their well-being in terms of emotion, connections, and meaning. More generally, in order to advance technologies' ability in this sense, it is important to consider motivational and emotional factors. Indeed, it is more frequent for users to use (even at a long term) technologies that are not easy to use but that they *love*, than the contrary. The following sections will explore motivation and emotional factors as important aspects to be considered both when evaluating and designing technology.

2.2.1 Motivation in Design

"Motivation" generally refers to any mental feature that guides and promotes human goal-directed behavior. Assessing motivation to use technology requires going beyond traditional conceptions of motivation that held that people give more value to strictly physical or safety needs, and only after satisfying them consider relational or self-actualizing motives (e.g., having friends, succeed in one's own passions, spirituality, etc.). On the contrary, depending on current situations and personal goals, people may put high-level needs before basic ones. According to Self Determination Theory (Ryan and Deci 2000), fundamental life "nutrients" regard creating and maintaining positive relationships with others, feeling competent and autonomous. Hassenzahl and colleagues (Hassenzahl et al. 2010) developed motivation-focused interviewees in order to consider users' important motivation when designing or evaluating products and artifacts. In the field of user-centered design for eHealth interventions, one should consider that users' needs may vary depending on the experience and perception of the long-lasting illness, and so do life projects and everyday activities (Triberti and Barello 2016). It is not advisable to design eHealth technologies just considering therapy outcomes and/or desired health states; on the contrary, if technologies are designed to be used effectively, they should be able to communicate their scope as useful in terms of patients' personal objectives (Triberti and Riva 2016).

2.2.2 Emotion in Design

"Emotional design" is an expression typically used to refer to that design which is implemented to promote a pleasurable sensation in users. Two main approaches can be found in the literature, one more focused on pleasant, funny, creative features added to interfaces or external appearance (Jordan 2002), and the other related to engaging and fluent interaction (Hancock et al. 2005). Recent studies (Triberti et al. 2017) proposed to develop the concept of emotional design through three main lines:

- The assessment of discrete emotions in ongoing interaction with technology to provide on-line modifications of interfaces (affective computing/affective design).
- The focus on emotions as discrete cognitive processes instead of generic pleasant states, to promote even complex emotions or emotional nuances.
- The analysis of users' "emotional profiles" to tailor technologies on their preexisting emotional traits.

In other words, emotions should not be considered as simply by-products of stimuli, rather they could actively participate in the interaction and influence it. Also, not only positive emotions should be taken into consideration by designers; for example, if one has to design a eHealth platform feature that is meant to signal dangerous situations to the patient (e.g., the need for insulin administration for diabetes), it is not expected to transform an urgent signal into a "positive" experience, which it is not. On the contrary, if previous emotion-focused research is available, designers and evaluators can have important information on how to realize such an alarm so to be recognized, understood, and managed as more effectively as possible by the patient/user.

Emotion aspects research can certainly be conducted by making use of psychophysiological measures, but also qualitative methods are important in order to capture the personal emotional experience of patients, regarding both the illness/ treatment experience and the technology itself.

2.3 Context

P5 eHealth must consider context as an important variable for UX and delivery of care. In particular, psycho-social aspects of the P5 approach are involved in this process. Any technological artifact related to eHealth, or otherwise, is made to be used by someone for a particular context, in a particular environment. The user's purpose guides the artifact's design first and later its use, which is situated in a precise space-time moment. The user experience is therefore—and perhaps above all—linked to the places and moments in which the user uses the artifact "in vivo." In this sense, for the purposes of the design and evaluation of the user experience, the context of use must be taken into account.

Context is a difficult concept to define and can indicate: material elements of the environment in which the use takes place; relational elements, when artifacts mediate the relationships between people directly or indirectly; and semiotic and cultural elements (Galimberti 2011). Several of these aspects must be taken into consideration in the design phase; others, on the other hand, are more unpredictable and emerge from the interaction between artifact–user–context (Nardi 1996), and once these aspects are detected, they could be corrected and/or integrated into subsequent releases of the artifact to improve the users' UX.

The Situated Action Theory (SAT) (Mantovani 1995, 1996; Suchman 1987, 1993) helps understand that behavior, cognition, and higher-level contextual elements, such as cultural, organizational, and group settings, contribute to the interactional process between user and technology—and thus affect UX—at different levels: context of use depends on social context, interpretation of the situation, and local interaction with artifacts. The first level, the social context, is seen as a repertoire of social norms, within which actors must act. The second level considers daily experience, where the social context refers to specific situations in which the interests of social actors interact with the opportunities presented by the environment. The last level relates to local interaction between man and artifact, which occurs in everyday situations, whenever the user uses the artifact to achieve their goals.

eHealth technologies are considered technological artifacts, therefore they are bound by cultural and social rules, the situation in which they are used, and by how the aims and scopes of the users interweave with the previously mentioned aspects and the material feature of the artifact itself (e.g., the interface).

Norman (1993) wrote that it is not enough to focus individually on the situation, artifact, environment, or person: the users are not in a vacuum, but are located in a specific context. The symbolic order is achieved through action, which allows the interpretation of the situation, which in turn allows actors to use certain artifacts in certain situations. Context is built on a cultural and symbolic order (rules, laws, social habits, cultural norms) that preexists the user in interaction, but also contributes to the users' activities and directs their goals: context helps the users make sense of their actions and interactions. Within a context, users are not alone, but interact with other actors and artifacts in order to accomplish their goals and plans. New meaning is generated by the interaction between subjects and artifacts. These meanings become part of and they partially modify the symbolic order, generating new meanings.

Material artifacts—such as objects, technologies, etc.—are readily available to people, but they are not exempt from important psychological and signification processes: if a technological artifact is inadequate for use within the rules governing the context, and does not meet the objectives of the users, it will produce an unsatisfactory user experience and will soon be abandoned; it is almost impossible to determine in advance in a univocal way the use that users will make of an artifact, it will therefore be necessary to carry out in-progress checks in order, if possible, to adapt the artifact to the emerging practices resulting from the interaction with social actors.

Robinson (1994) postulated the existence of three reference frameworks that people use to interpret artifacts. This interpretative process involves a user's assumption, knowledge, bias, and past experiences shaping their understanding of the world. There are three frameworks that drive this process (Robinson 1994): (a) individual level: frameworks constitute, at this level, personal constructs: our way of being has an influence on the way we interface with and interpret the world; (b) social level: our interpretative schemes are built with the people we interact with, in the different contexts (e.g., work, family) and these references also contribute to our understanding of artifacts; (c) cultural level: this level refers to language, religion, visions of science and the world, conceptions of space and time (e.g., seasons, cyclicality), which permeate our way of interacting with people and objects around us.

In conclusion, context can be defined by three dimensions that can be ascribed to both Robinson's frameworks and to the Situated Action Theory: individual and psycho-social aspects, cultural and relational aspects, material/physical aspects. The following paragraphs outline each of these dimensions and how eHealth may be affected.

2.3.1 Individual and Psychosocial Dimensions of Context

Gender, age, and culture are aspects that affect the user's acceptance—in terms of adoption and speed of adoption—of technological artifacts. The Technology Acceptance Model (TAM) (Davis 1989) theorizes the process from the user's intention to use the technology to its final adoption. The TAM explains the intention to use an artifact on the basis of perceived utility (i.e., the perception of obtaining a benefit from the use of that artifact) and perceived ease of use (i.e., the perception that using that artifact will require few resources). If there is a high level of perceived utility and a high level of perceived ease of use, the user will be likely to develop the intention to adopt that particular artifact. External variables such as system characteristics, training, etc. do not affect directly on the intention to adopt the system, but their effect is mediated by the two variables previously explained.

Utility is influenced by perceived ease of use: the easier the artifact is to use, the more useful it is perceived to be (Venkatesh and Davis 2000). More recently, other factors have been added as antecedents to the intention of adoption and to the variables of perceived utility and ease of use, such as social influence (subjective norms, image, etc.), cognitive processes (relevance of the task, quality of the outputs, demonstrability of the results), and experience (Venkatesh and Davis 2000).

There are clear differences in gender with regard to the TAM. Venkatesh and Morris (2000) found that men and women differ in decision-making processes for adoption and use of technologies (cf. Chap. 4); in particular, the perceived user-friendliness variable is more important for women, despite identical initial training and identical experience with technology.

Men and women also differ in access and use, interest and ease of use of technological artifacts (Anderson et al. 1995), even though this gap is rapidly closing. One of the most important gender differences is related to the perceived self-efficacy (Bandura 1997) in the use of technologies, that is, the belief of being able to use a technology to perform a certain action (Durndell and Haag 2002; Vekiri and Chronaki 2008): in particular, even in the simple use of computers, males, compared to females, feel more secure and able to address the problems that may arise during the use of technology in a flexible and creative way (Brivio and Ibarra 2010). It can therefore be assumed that in the event of a technology breakdown, men and women will have very different experiences, and experience different emotions, with effects on their self-esteem and self-efficacy. The processes of breakdown and consequent troubleshooting for the recovery of technology functionality should probably be investigated in more detail from a gender point of view, to make them more accessible to all. In other respects, the user experience between men and women does not differ, although there are sometimes artifacts that try to exaggerate these differences. Self-efficacy (along with the variables of TAM) affects the use of technologies by older people, who have never had to deal with complex technologies (e.g., smartphone and tablet), and often do not feel confident in interacting with these artifacts, which very often are not designed with the elderly in mind, which makes the interaction difficult and the experience sometimes frustrating (Brivio et al. 2016; Strada et al. 2013).

Research with eHealth technologies show that age can still impact adoption and use, especially with middle-old (66–84 year olds) and old-old (85 years and over) people, who need more training and support (Hunsaker and Hargittai 2018; Millard and Fintak 2002); only after training and support are they more likely to adopt and use eHealth systems, as the interactional experience is less frustrating. Young old people (55–65 year old) have fewer issues with use and adoption (Tavares and Oliveira 2016). The gender gap in eHealth adoption seems to be slowly closing (Tavares and Oliveira 2016). A variable specific to adoption and use of eHealth technologies is self-perception, that is, the awareness of having a health problem: if a person is aware that they have a health issue they are more likely to use eHealth technologies (Tavares and Oliveira 2016; Yuan et al. 2015; Venkatesh et al. 2012). eHealth applications and technologies should therefore include in-system trainings for target populations, and enhance self-perception, in order to provide a good UX, which in turn ensures higher levels of intention to use, adoption, and sustained use.

2.3.2 Cultural and Relational Dimensions of Context

A cultural aspect that influences the User Experience is the semiotic dimension that underlies the artifacts. Semiotics deals with the study of signs and how they take on meaning. Every aspect of an interface can be considered a representation of a certain functionality to which it gives access: both the interface and the functionality to which it refers are systems of signs (Goguen 1999). Sustained use of an artifact depends on the user's understanding of the metaphor underlying the design of an artifact (Barr et al. 2005): designers must choose a sign system that helps the user understand the artifact's functionalities. If there is no correspondence between the systems of signs of the artifact and that of the user, the artifact will not be understandable and will provide an insufficient UX.

The most general distinction between cultural contexts that has proved to be relevant to UX is the one between Western and Eastern, individualistic or collectivistic cultures. Culture is "the collective programming of the mind that distinguishes the members of one group from another" (Hofstede 1991, 2001): the term "collective planning of the mind" suggests that culture can be conceived as a set of shared characteristics within a group, whose members behave similarly because of the shared norms. User Experience is also influenced by these shared characteristics: for an artifact to be successful at an international level, it is necessary to have an excellent knowledge of the variability of the cultures of the target markets, since sometimes an international version of an artifact may not be sufficient or may not work at all in terms of needs and cultural appropriateness (Marcus and Gould 2000). To have artifacts that adapt to different cultures, two aspects must be taken into account (Honold 1999, in Walsh et al. 2010): (1) objective aspects: language, date and time format, numbers, direction of written text, etc.; (2) subjective aspects: value, behavioral, and intellectual systems of the groups that use technological artifacts in the different cultural contexts. These aspects can be integrated into the design of artifacts from the beginning, using the studies and tables (created by country) of Hofstede (1991), taking into account that the indications given are always trends and always relative. Not all aspects of interaction with a technological artifact are, however, subject to cultural differences: for example, it seems that gestures—spontaneously generated to obtain a result on a portable device—are not culturally connoted and resemble each other for all cultures (Mauney et al. 2010).

To provide excellent UX and delivery of care, eHealth technologies and application must take these aspects into consideration, and go through a cultural and contextual adaptation process for "culturally sensitive elements" (e.g., language, values, concepts, content) (Lal et al. 2018). For the relational dimension—as Battarbee points out (2003)—the User Experience models used often focus on individual experience and its constituent elements; most people though experience collective, not individual, contexts and thus create experiences with artifacts together with other users (Battarbee 2003, 2004; Battarbee and Koskinen 2005). Artifacts must of course be functional, usable, and provide a good individual user experience; but, with the advent of personal ICT, it is important that these artifacts give users the opportunity to have optimal user experiences together, or to have a co-experience. Battarbee identifies some characteristics that the co-experience given by an artifact must have:

- Social: co-experience is based on communication, which allows proposals, opinions, evaluations to be put into play, agreements to be negotiated, ideas modified, etc. These communicative exchanges give meaning to the experience. It is therefore essential that the artifacts support agile communication exchanges and that they reflect the communication needs of users in a given context.
- Multimodal: co-experience can be augmented by technology, which provides different modes of interaction (e.g., audio, video, image, text) and allows switching between them seamlessly, while continuing to have the same experience with the same people or with different people.
- Creative: when people use technological artifacts together, they get more interesting and creative results than those obtained with individual use. Co-experience is a resource of social and symbolic innovation, because interaction generates new meanings, both related to technology and not.
- Fun: co-experience is a source of fun and pleasure, as well as it strengthens social ties. Fun promotes the use of artifacts. For designers, therefore, it is essential to think about the dimension of enjoyment and pleasure in social terms, because it is a fundamental motivation for the adoption and sustained use of an artifact.

Any environment that involves co-presence of multiple people needs individuals to feel that the other is present: in other words, to perceive a good sense of social presence, which is "the degree of salience of the other person in the interaction and the consequent salience of the interpersonal relationship" (Short et al. 1976). An adequate level of social presence allows higher levels of involvement with the artifact, that is, the user experience will be more satisfying and positive (Gunawardena and Zittle 1997). According to Riva and colleagues (2008), social presence depends on the fact that the information available within the context, even if limited, allows the users to grasp the others' intentions and actions (Riva 2008).

In eHealth, several technologies and applications successfully harnessed social communications and exchange between users to deliver their intervention, for example in smoking cessation (Khalil et al. 2017) and in psychosis recovery (Williams et al. 2018). This made possible not only delivery of care, but also a good UX that could potentially support adherence and sustained use of the eHealth system.

2.3.3 Physical and Material Dimension of Context

In designing or evaluating an artifact, technological or otherwise, it is important to know where the user will use the artifact itself. The physical environment produces effects on UX in different ways. For example, placement of a technology within a busy and noisy environment may influence the user's ability to hear acoustic feedback (Lowdermilk 2013). Mobile technologies complicate this matter further: they allow user to cross different contexts; and indeed, the use of some applications persists from one context—digital and material—to another, and therefore the experience persists across contexts, and designers must take these contextual changes into consideration.

Literature is lacking in identifying and describing the effect of the physical contextual elements on eHealth delivery and UX. One possible concern is related to privacy: mHealth makes it easier to access health services and care, but at the same time make it easier for private and sensitive information to be available, accessible or overheard by non-authorized people, or to use the technology in inappropriate settings for delivery of care (e.g., a patient using a telepsychotherapy service in a public setting). Consequence of accidental sharing of information and/or use in appropriate settings may be an inefficient delivery of care and/or a reduced UX, which in turn may push people to abandon the eHealth service.

3 User-Centered Design and P5 eHealth

As hinted at in the introduction, User-Centered Design should be a fundamental methodological approach within P5 eHealth: in order to design health technologies that are really able to help people, it is paramount to analyze users/patients' needs, intentions, abilities, and contexts in advance, and use these data as the main source for design ideas and implementation.

As a conclusion, it is interesting to consider the utility of a UCD mindset when designing the P5 properties within health technologies:

- For designing technologies with **prevention** features, developers should be informed not only about healthy behaviors to be promoted in the users, but also of users' own habits, preferences, characteristics, and typical behaviors in order to identify risks and/or opportunities.
- **Personalized** technology requires up-to-date information about users' characteristics; the exact concept of personalization of application features implies to consider and understand users, instead of basing on prototypical representations.
- The **predictive** power of any computational model programmed within software is notably empowered by adding information on users' preferences and behaviors; not only medical/diagnostical data should be used.
- **Participatory** technologies require a deep understanding of users' social context; going beyond the mere analysis of users, methods should be able to capture important social relations (e.g., caregivers, different health professionals) to be assigned a role within the technology-based intervention.
- **Psycho-cognitive** technologies, as previously said, are able to consider users' cognitive abilities, decision making, and behavior; this could be done by implementing the UCD mindset/approach within the technology itself, which means, the technology should be responsive to users' actions in order to tailor its outcomes (feedback) on individual characteristics.

With this background, P5 eHealth could develop as a truly patient-centered approach, by basing its own design on the application of research methods to the measurement and understanding of final users' irreducible characteristics.

References

Abras, C., Maloney-krichmar, D., & Preece, J. (2004). User-centered design. In *Encyclopedia of human-computer interaction* (pp. 1–14). New York: Sage.

Anderson, R., Bikson, T., Law, S., & Mitchell, B. (1995). *Universal access to e-mail: Feasibility and social implications*. Main: RAND Corporation.

Bandura, A. (1997). *Self-efficacy: The exercise of control*. New York: W H Freeman/Times Books/ Henry Holt & Co..

Barr, P., Biddle, R., & Noble, J. (2005). A semiotic model of user-interface metaphor. In K. Liu (Ed.), *Virtual, distributed and flexible organisations* (pp. 189–215). Dordrecht: Springer. https://doi.org/10.1007/1-4020-2162-3_13.

Battarbee, K. (2003). Co-experience: The social user experience. *CHI 2003 Extended Abstracts on Human Factors in Computing Systems*, 730–731. https://doi.org/10.1145/765891.765956.

Battarbee, K. (2004). *Co-experience: Understanding user experiences in social interaction*. Helsinki: UIAH Press.

Battarbee, K., & Koskinen, I. (2005). Co-experience: User experience as interaction. *CoDesign, 1*(1), 5–18. https://doi.org/10.1080/15710880412331289917.

Benyon, D., Turner, P., & Turner, S. (2005). *Designing interactive systems: People, activities, contexts, technologies*. Addison-Wesley. Retrieved from https://books.google.com/books?id= iWe7VkFW0zMC&pgis=1.

Brivio, E., & Ibarra, F. C. (2010). Nuove Tecnologie e Autoefficacia percepita: Influenze del genere e delle modalità d' uso. *Qwerty, 5*(1), 44–59.

Brivio, E., Serino, S., Galimberti, C., & Riva, G. (2016). Efficacy of a digital education program on Life Satisfaction and digital self efficacy: A mixed method study. *Annual Review of Cybertherapy and Telemedicine*.

Brooke, J. (1996). SUS - A quick and dirty usability scale. In P. Jordan, B. Thomas, B. McClelland, & I. Weerdmeester (Eds.), *Usability evaluation in industry* (pp. 189–194). London: Taylor & Francis. https://doi.org/10.1002/hbm.20701.

Davis, F. D. (1989). Perceived usefulness, perceived ease of use, and user acceptance of information technology. *MIS Quarterly, 13*(3), 319. https://doi.org/10.2307/249008.

Durndell, A., & Haag, Z. (2002). Computer self efficacy, computer anxiety, attitudes towards the Internet and reported experience with the Internet, by gender, in an East European sample. *Computers in Human Behavior, 18*(5), 521–535. https://doi.org/10.1016/ S0747-5632(02)00006-7.

Galimberti, C. (2011). Segui il coniglio bianco: La costruzione della soggettività nelle interazioni mediate. In E. Marta & C. Regalia (Eds.), *Identità in Relazione: Le sfide odierne dell'essere adulto* (pp. 73–127). Milano: McGraw-Hill.

Garrett, J. J. (2010). *The elements of user experience: User-centered design for the web and beyond*. (Pearson Ed). Pearson Education.

Gerdes, M., Smaradottir, B., & Fensli, R. (2014). End-to-end infrastructure for usability evaluation of eHealth applications and services. *Scandinavian Conference on Health Informatics, 53*.

Goguen, J. (1999). An introduction to algebraic semiotics, with applications to user interface design. *Computation for Metaphors, Analogy and Agents*, 242–291.

Goldberg, L., Lide, B., Lowry, S., Massett, H. A., O'Connell, T., Preece, J., et al. (2011). Usability and accessibility in consumer health informatics: Current trends and future challenges. *American Journal of Preventive Medicine, 40*(5 SUPPL. 2), S187–S197. https://doi. org/10.1016/j.amepre.2011.01.009.

Gorini, A., & Pravettoni, G. (2011). P5 medicine: A plus for a personalized approach to oncology. *Nature Reviews Clinical Oncology*. https://doi.org/10.1038/nrclinonc.2010.227-c1.

Gunawardena, C. N., & Zittle, F. J. (1997). Social presence as a predictor of satisfaction within a computer-mediated conferencing environment. *American Journal of Distance Education, 11*(3), 8–26. https://doi.org/10.1080/08923649709526970.

Hancock, P. A., Pepe, A., & Murphy, L. L. (2005). Hedonomics: The power of positive and pleasurable ergonomics. *Design, 13*, 8–14. https://doi.org/10.1177/106480460501300104.

Hassenzahl, M. (2008). User experience (UX): Towards an experiential perspective on product quality. In *IHM'08* (pp. 11–15). https://doi.org/10.1145/1512714.1512717.
Hassenzahl, M., Diefenbach, S., & Göritz, A. (2010). Needs, affect, and interactive products–Facets of user experience. *Interacting with computers, 22*(5), 353–362.
Hermawati, S., & Lawson, G. (2016). Establishing usability heuristics for heuristics evaluation in a specific domain: Is there a consensus? *Applied ergonomics, 56*, 34–51.
Herstatt, C., & Von Hippel, E. A. (1992). From experience: Developing new product concepts via the lead user method: A case study in a "low tech" field. *Journal of Product Innovation Management.* https://doi.org/10.1016/0737-6782(92)90031-7.
Hesse, B. W., & Shneiderman, B. (2007). eHealth research from the user's perspective. *American Journal of Preventive Medicine, 32*(5 Suppl). https://doi.org/10.1016/j.amepre.2007.01.019.
Hofstede, G. H. (1991). *Cultures and organizations: Software of the mind.* McGraw-Hill.
Hofstede, G. H. (2001). *Culture's consequences: Comparing values, behaviors, institutions, and organizations across nations.* Sage.
Hunsaker, A., & Hargittai, E. (2018). A review of Internet use among older adults. *New Media & Society, 20*(10), 3937–3954. https://doi.org/10.1177/1461444818787348.
Jordan, P. W. (2002). *Designing pleasurable products—An induction to the new human factors.* London: Taylor and Francis.
Karwowski, W. (2012). The discipline of human factors and ergonomics. In G. Salvendy (Ed.), *Handbook of human factors and ergonomics.* New York: Wiley. https://doi.org/10.1002/0470048204.ch27.
Khalil, G. E., Wang, H., Calabro, K. S., Mitra, N., Shegog, R., & Prokhorov, A. V. (2017). From the experience of interactivity and entertainment to lower intention to smoke: A randomized controlled trial and path analysis of a web-based smoking prevention program for adolescents. *Journal of Medical Internet Research, 19*(2), e44. https://doi.org/10.2196/jmir.7174.
Kushniruk, A. W., Monkman, H., Tuden, D., Bellwood, P., & Borycki, E. M. (2015). Integrating heuristic evaluation with cognitive walkthrough: Development of a hybrid usability inspection method. *Studies in Health Technology and Informatics, 208*, 221–225.
Lal, S., Gleeson, J., Malla, A., Rivard, L., Joober, R., Chandrasena, R., & Alvarez-Jimenez, M. (2018). Cultural and contextual adaptation of an eHealth intervention for youth receiving services for first-episode psychosis: Adaptation framework and protocol for horyzons-canada phase 1. *JMIR Research Protocols, 7*(4), e100. https://doi.org/10.2196/resprot.8810.
Lee, I., Choi, G. W., Kim, J., Kim, S., Lee, K., Kim, D., ... & An, Y. (2008, September). *Cultural dimensions for user experience: cross-country and cross-product analysis of users' cultural characteristics.* In Proceedings of the 22nd British HCI Group Annual Conference on People and Computers: Culture, Creativity, Interaction-Volume 1 (pp. 3–12). British Computer Society.
Lowdermilk, T. (2013). *User-centered design: A developer's guide to building userfFriendly applications.* Sebastopol: O'Reilly.
Mantovani, G. (1995). *Comunicazione e identità : dalle situazioni quotidiane agli ambienti virtuali.* Il mulino.
Mantovani, G. (1996). Social context in HCl: A new framework for mental models, cooperation, and communication. *Cognitive Science, 20*(2), 237–269. https://doi.org/10.1207/s15516709cog2002_3.
Marcus, A., & Gould, E. W. (2000). Crosscurrents: Cultural dimensions and global Web user-interface design. *Interactions, 7*(4), 32–46. https://doi.org/10.1145/345190.345238.
Mauney, D., Howarth, J., Wirtanen, A., & Capra, M. (2010). Cultural similarities and differences in user-defined gestures for touchscreen user interfaces. In *Extended abstracts of the 28th international conference on human factors in computing systems (CHI'10)* (pp. 4015–4020). https://doi.org/10.1145/1753846.1754095.
Millard, R. W., & Fintak, P. A. (2002). Use of the internet by patients with chronic illness. *Disease Management and Health Outcomes, 10*(3), 187–194. https://doi.org/10.2165/00115677-200210030-00006.
Nardi, B. A. (1996). *Context and consciousness: Activity theory and human-computer interaction.* MIT Press.

Nickerson, R. (1999). Chapter 1 - Engineering psychology and ergonomics. In P. Hancock (Ed.), *Human performance and ergonomics*. https://doi.org/10.1016/B978-012322735-5/50002-6.
Nielsen, J. (1995). 10 usability heuristics for user interface design. *Nielsen Norman Group, 1*(1).
Nielsen, J. (1999). User interface directions for the Web. *Communications of the ACM*. https://doi.org/10.1145/291469.291470.
Nielsen, J. (2003). Usability 101: Introduction to usability. *All Usability, 9*, 1–10.
Norman, D. A. (2002). The design of everyday things. Human factors and ergonomics in manufacturing (Vol. 16). Basic Books. doi:https://doi.org/10.1002/hfm.20127
Norman, D. A., & Draper, S. W. (1986). *User centered system design: New perspectives on human-computer interaction*. Lawrence Erlbaum Associates.
Pavelin, K., Cham, J. A., de Matos, P., Brooksbank, C., Cameron, G., & Steinbeck, C. (2012). Bioinformatics meets user-centred design: A perspective. *PLoS Computational Biology*. https://doi.org/10.1371/journal.pcbi.1002554.
Pravettoni, G., & Gorini, A. (2011). A P5 cancer medicine approach: Why personalized medicine cannot ignore psychology. *Journal of Evaluation in Clinical Practice, 17*(4), 594–596. https://doi.org/10.1111/j.1365-2753.2011.01709.x.
Riva, G. (2008). Enacting interactivity: The role of presence. In F. Morganti, A. Carassa, & G. Riva (Eds.), *Enacting intersubjecitvity: A cognitive and social perspective on the study of interactions* (pp. 97–114). Amsterdam: IOS press.
Riva, G., Villani, D., Cipresso, P., Repetto, C., Triberti, S., Di Lernia, D., et al. (2016). Positive and transformative technologies for active ageing. *Studies in Health Technology and Informatics, 220*, 308.
Robinson, R. E. (1994). Making sense of making sense: Frameworks and organizational perception. *Design Management Journal, 5*(1), 8–15. https://doi.org/10.1111/j.1948-7169.1994.tb00611.x.
Ryan, R. M., & Deci, E. L. (2000). Self-determination theory and the facilitation of intrinsic motivation, social development, and well-being. *American Psychologist, 55*(1), 68.
Sharit, J. (2006). Human error. In G. Salvendy (Ed.), *Handbook of human factors and ergonomics*. https://doi.org/10.1002/0470048204.ch27.
Short, J., Williams, E., & Christie, B. (1976). *The social psychology of telecommunications*. Wiley.
Smilowitz, E. D., Darnell, M. J., & Benson, A. E. (1994). Are we overlooking some usability testing methods? A comparison of lab, beta, and forum tests. *Behaviour & Information Technology, 13*(1-2), 183–190.
Strada, C., Brivio, E., & Galimberti, C. (2013). Digital education for older generation non native users: a focused ethnography study of a pilot project. *Qwerty-Open and Interdisciplinary Journal of Technology, Culture and Education, 8*(2), 44–57.
Suchman, L. A. (1987). *Plans and situated actions: The problem of human-machine communication*. New York: Cambridge University Press.
Suchman, L. (1993). Response to vera and simon's situated action: A symbolic interpretation. *Cognitive Science, 17*(1), 71–75. https://doi.org/10.1207/s15516709cog1701_5.
Tavares, J., & Oliveira, T. (2016). Electronic health record patient portal adoption by health care consumers: An acceptance model and survey. *Journal of Medical Internet Research, 18*(3), e49. https://doi.org/10.2196/jmir.5069.
Triberti, S., & Barello, S. (2016). The quest for engaging AmI: Patient engagement and experience design tools to promote effective assisted living. *Journal of Biomedical Informatics, 63*. https://doi.org/10.1016/j.jbi.2016.08.010.
Triberti, S., & Brivio, E. (2017). *User experience*. Milan: Maggioli.
Triberti, S., & Liberati, E. G. (2014). Patient centered virtual reality: An opportunity to improve the quality of patient's experience. In P. Cipresso & S. Serino (Eds.), *Virtual reality: Technologies, medical applications and challenges*. Nova Science.
Triberti, S., & Riva, G. (2016). Being present in action: a theoretical model about the "interlocking" between intentions and environmental affordances. *Frontiers in Psychology, 6*, 2052.

Triberti, S., Chirico, A., La Rocca, G., & Riva, G. (2017). Developing emotional design: Emotions as cognitive processes and their role in the design of interactive technologies. *Frontiers in Psychology, 8*, 1773.

Vekiri, I., & Chronaki, A. (2008). Gender issues in technology use: Perceived social support, computer self-efficacy and value beliefs, and computer use beyond school. *Computers and Education, 51*(3), 1392–1404. https://doi.org/10.1016/j.compedu.2008.01.003.

Venkatesh, V., & Davis. (2000). A theoretical extension of the technology acceptance model: Four longitudinal field studies. *Management Science, 46*(2), 186–204. https://doi.org/10.1287/mnsc.46.2.186.11926.

Venkatesh, V., & Morris, M. G. (2000). Why don' t men ever stop to ask for directions? Gender, social influence, and their role in technology acceptance and usage behavior. *MIS Quarterly, 24*(1), 115–139.

Vergani, L., Marton, G., Pizzoli, S. F. M., Monzani, D., Mazzocco, K., & Pravettoni, G. (2019). Training cognitive functions using mobile apps in breast cancer patients: Systematic review. *JMIR mHealth and uHealth, 7*(3), e10855.

Vorderstrasse, A., Lewinski, A., Melkus, G. D., & Johnson, C. (2016). Social support for diabetes self-management via eHealth interventions. *Current Diabetes Reports.* https://doi.org/10.1007/s11892-016-0756-0.

Walsh, T., Nurkka, P., & Walsh, R. (2010). Cultural differences in smartphone user experience evaluation. *Mum'10.*

Williams, A., Fossey, E., Farhall, J., Foley, F., & Thomas, N. (2018). Recovery after psychosis: Qualitative study of service user experiences of lived experience videos on a recovery-oriented website. *JMIR Mental Health, 5*(2), e37. https://doi.org/10.2196/mental.9934.

Wilson, J. R. (2000). Fundamentals of ergonomics in theory and practice. *Applied Ergonomics, 31*(6), 557–567. https://doi.org/10.1016/S0003-6870(00)00034-X.

Yuan, S., Ma, W., Kanthawala, S., & Peng, W. (2015). Keep using my health apps: Discover users' perception of health and fitness apps with the UTAUT2 model. *Telemedicine and E-Health, 21*(9), 735–741. https://doi.org/10.1089/tmj.2014.01.

Norman, D. A. (1993). Cognition in the head and in the world: An introduction to the special issue on situated action. *Cognitive Science, 17*(1), 1–6.

Venkatesh, V., Thong, J. Y., & Xu, X. (2012). Consumer acceptance and use of information technology: Extending the unified theory of acceptance and use of technology. *MIS Quarterly, 36*(1), 157–178.

Chapter 10
Data Protection and Ethical Issues in European P5 eHealth

Virginia Sanchini and Luca Marelli

1 Introduction

In spite of its promise to significantly ameliorate health and care practices, the momentous rise of eHealth technologies—an umbrella term that refers to a varied set of tools and resources such as health information networks, electronic health records, telemedicine and monitoring services, wearable systems, as well as online health self-management tools—has been fraught with significant ethical and societal concerns. Thriving out of the extensive use of (sensitive) personal data (i.e., Big Data approach), while also representing a major driver for reconfiguring entrenched social practices and relations within health and care systems, eHealth has been the focus, in recent years, of increased ethical, legal, and sociological scrutiny.

Aimed at providing an overview of the data protection regime and the main ethical issues associated with the emergence and progressive stabilization of eHealth within the context of the European Union (EU), this chapter is structured as follows. First, innovation in eHealth as a core policy objective of the EU is presented; then, regulatory issues related to eHealth research and innovation are discussed; notably, our attention will be devoted to the discussion of eHealth technologies in light of the

The Authors Virginia Sanchini and Luca Marelli have contributed equally to this work.

V. Sanchini (✉)
Faculty of Philosophy, Università Vita-Salute San Raffaele, Milan, Italy

Department of Oncology and Hemato-Oncology, University of Milan, Milan, Italy
e-mail: sanchini.virginia@hsr.it; virginia.sanchini@unimi.it

L. Marelli
Life Sciences & Society Lab, Centre for Sociological Research, KU Leuven, Belgium

Department of Experimental Oncology, IEO, European Institute of Oncology IRCCS, Milan, Italy
e-mail: luca.marelli@kuleuven.be; luca.marelli@ieo.it

G. Pravettoni, S. Triberti (eds.), *P5 eHealth: An Agenda for the Health Technologies of the Future*, https://doi.org/10.1007/978-3-030-27994-3_10

regulatory regime unfolding in Europe following the enforceability of the new legislation on data protection, Regulation (EU) 2016/679, also known as the General Data Protection Regulation. Finally, the second part of the chapter will provide an overview of the main ethical challenges raised by the development and implementation of novel eHealth technologies.

2 eHealth in the European Union: From Advancement of Innovation to Data Protection Concerns

Ever increasingly since the launch of the Lisbon Agenda at the turn of the millennium, the European Union (EU) has targeted the acceleration of scientific and technological innovation as a key policy objective. Emphasized as one of the privileged means to steer the EU out of its current economic and political gridlock, the acceleration of innovation has also been envisaged as a prominent lever to relaunch the promise of the European project and to promote the further consolidation of the fragile European polity (Marelli and Testa 2017).

Notably, innovation in eHealth, which thrives out of advances in fields such as personalized medicine, Artificial Intelligence, Big Data Analytics and mobile Health (mHealth) technologies, has emerged, in recent years, as a major recipient of knowledge and material investments from the part of the Union, geared to "strengthen[ing] the resilience and sustainability of Europe's health and care systems" and "maximiz[ing] the potential of the digital internal market with a wider deployment of digital products and services" (EC 2018: 4). Specifically, the latest Communication from the European Commission on *Enabling the digital transformation of health and care in the Digital Single Market* (EC 2018) has identified three key objectives to be accomplished through the full-fledged digitization of health and care systems and the (yet-to-be-achieved) completion of the Digital Single Market—a policy cornerstone of the European Commission under the presidency of Jean-Claude Juncker—in the health and care domains.

Firstly, the Commission set out its intention to enhance the sharing of health data across borders, by "supporting the development and adoption of a European electronic health record exchange format" (EC 2018, p. 5), predicated on the interoperability of standards across Member States, the development of EU-wide standards for data quality, reliability and cybersecurity, as well as potential (re)use of data for research and other purposes. A second envisaged objective is represented by the "pooling of genomic and other health data to advance research and personalized medicine" (EC 2018, p. 7). Specifically, against the backdrop of a flurry of initiatives having mushroomed throughout European Member States in recent years, the EU is tasked with "linking national and regional banks of -omics data, biobanks and other registries," with the aim of "provid[ing] access to at least 1 million sequenced genomes in the EU by 2022" (EC 2018, p. 8). Thirdly—and most relevantly for the purposes of this chapter—the digitization of health and care through the integration of eHealth technologies and practices in health and care systems is framed as directed toward the enactment of "citizen empowerment and person-centered care" (EC 2018, p. 10). Indeed, ageing of the population together with the growing burden of chronic conditions and multi-morbidity are said to require profound changes in health and care systems (cf. Chap. 1). As contended by the Commission, what is required is, in particular, a "shift from treatment to health promotion and disease prevention, from focus to disease to a focus on well-being and individuals, and from service fragmentation to the integration and coordination of services along the continuum of care" (EC 2018, p. 10).

Notwithstanding the emphasis placed on the advancement of innovation in the eHealth sector, poised to the creation of a "Europe-wide ecosystem for data-driven healthcare" (Smith 2018), EU policymakers have been equally alerted to the privacy and data protection concerns European citizens maintain when confronted with these new technologies and practices (Mager 2017). Accordingly, following trilogue (and extensively lobbied) negotiations started in 2012, in 2016 the European Parliament has approved Regulation (EU) 2016/679 on data protection, also known as the General Data Protection Regulation (GDPR). As remarked by its rapporteur, German MEP Jan Albrecht, the GDPR is intended to provide "the right balance between the fundamental right to data protection as well as strong consumer rights in the digital age, on the one side, and the need to create a fair and functioning digital market, with a real chance for growth and innovation, on the other side" (Albrecht 2016).

In what follows, we will explore the impact of the GDPR on the European eHealth sector. In particular, our focus is directed at charting some of the key provisions of the GDPR that affect research and innovation processes in the eHealth sector. Besides, we will probe the implications of the Regulation as to the balancing of the interests and fundamental rights of individuals and the advancement of eHealth innovation.

3 The GDPR and Its Impact on eHealth Research and Innovation

The GDPR, which repeals the previous European legislation on data protection, Directive 95/46/EC, has become applicable since May 25, 2018. Differently from the previous Directive, which required adoption in national legislations, the GDPR is directly enforceable across all Member States, and is thus geared to achieve immediate and thorough legislative harmonization across the EU. Besides providing regulatory support for the establishment of a full-fledged digital single market, its entry into effect is bound to impact the eHealth sector very significantly, in the EU and possibly beyond. How, and to what effect, is what we aim to chart in the following sections.

At its core, as enshrined in the "data protection by design and by default" principle (art. 25), the GDPR adopts a risk-based approach to data protection, geared to ensure that appropriate data protection measures are designed and implemented throughout the entirety of the data processing activities. Additionally, it confers novel rights to data subjects, such as the right to data portability (art. 20) and the so-called right to be forgotten (art. 17). While the former bestows on individuals the right to require that data concerning them be standardized and made portable across companies or service providers of their choice, the latter empowers data subjects to obtain from data controllers the prompt erasure of relevant personal data. Moreover, the GDPR prescribes the adoption of specific provisions for the processing of sensitive data (art. 9) for scientific research purposes (art. 89), such as technical and organizational measures (e.g., pseudonymization), which are meant to provide adequate safeguards to the rights and freedoms of data subjects. Such provisions—which we will explore more in detail below—are poised to have a great impact on the development and commercialization of novel eHealth tools and technologies. Relevantly, the GDPR also endows Member States with the prerogative to maintain or introduce further conditions, including limitations, with regard to the processing of genetic data, biometric data or data concerning health (art. 9(4)).

3.1 The Accountability Principle and its Implications

In general terms, the axiomatic cornerstone of the GDPR can be said to be represented by the "accountability principle" (art. 5(2), art. 24), which requires data controllers (i.e., the persons, companies, associations, or other entities that are factually in control of personal-data processing) to adopt a proactive approach toward data protection compliance. Notably, data controllers are made responsible to assess, implement, and verify the adoption of appropriate technical and organizational measures to ensure, and be able to demonstrate, that data processing complies with the GDPR (art. 24). The GDPR itself provides coarse-grained guidance as to what measures actually fulfill a controller's obligations, and in fact makes the determination of those measures dependent on the contingent "nature, scope, context and purposes" of the relevant processing (art. 24). Accordingly, it can be argued that the GDPR is bound to promote a "controller-based," "case-sensitive," and eminently "context–specific" approach to data protection (Marelli and Testa 2018).

Such decentralized, flexible, and accountability-based approach rises to significance with respect to two aspects that are of key importance in the development and adoption phase of eHealth technologies, namely, consent and secondary use of data (further processing). With regard to consent, the GDPR requires the "specific [and] informed" consent of the data subject (art. 6(1)(a) and recital 32). However, when it comes to the processing of personal data within research—as can be the case in the developmental phase of eHealth technologies, such as mHealth apps, telemedical or Ambient Intelligence tools—it recognizes that it may not be possible to fully identify all potential future research purposes at the time of data collection. Accordingly, as per recital 33, it states that, if too specific a consent would impinge on the purpose of research, "data subjects should be allowed to give their consent to certain areas of scientific research when in keeping with recognized ethical standards for scientific research." Otherwise put, such provision lends the full legislative weight of the GDPR in support of broad consent, whenever the criterion of specific consent for specific research use at the moment of data collection proves impossible to satisfy (Marelli and Testa 2018).

As for the further use of previously collected and processed data—a key requirement for Big Data processing—article 5(1)(b) of the GDPR mandates that personal data should be "collected for specified, explicit and legitimate purposes and not further processed in a manner that is incompatible with those purposes." Additionally, it specifies that further processing for scientific research purposes "shall [...] not be considered to be incompatible with the initial purposes" for which personal data have been collected. More specifically, the GDPR requires controllers to carry out, on a case-by-case and context-dependent basis, a "test" for compatibility assessment, geared at ascertaining whether the further processing of personal data without data subject's consent is compatible with the initial purpose for which data were originally collected (art. 6(4)). Factors such as the "the reasonable expectations of data subjects based on their relationship with the controller as to their further use" (recital 50), and "the context in which the personal data have been collected," are among the key elements to be taken into account for assessing the compatibility of the intended further processing (art. 6(4)).

3.2 *Pseudonymization and Anonymization of Sensitive Data*

An important distinction introduced by the GDPR is the one between pseudonymized and anonymous data. Art. 4(5) defines "pseudonymization" as "*the processing of personal data in such a manner that the personal data can no longer be attributed to a specific data subject without the use of additional information, provided that such additional information is kept separately and is subject to technical and organizational measures to ensure that the personal data are not attributed to an identified or identifiable natural person.*" On the contrary, anonymous data are defined, as per recital 26, as "*information which does not relate to an identified or identifiable natural person or to personal data rendered anonymous in such a manner that the data subject is not or no longer identifiable.*" This difference has significant implications. On the one hand, pseudonymized data—insofar as they can be attributed to the data subject through the use of "additional information"—are considered as personal data whose processing should comply with the GDPR. On the other hand, the provisions of the GDPR "do not concern the processing of anonymous information, including for statistical or research purposes" (recital 26). In other words, whereas the processing of pseudonymized information should be subjected to the full spectrum of provisions contained in the GDPR, individuals will not be entitled to data protection rights if their data are processed anonymously.

But what does constitute "anonymous" processing (or, better phrased, processing of "anonymous" data) in light of the GDPR? Interestingly, the GDPR differs conspicuously, in this respect, from other major data protection legislations worldwide, such as the Health Insurance Portability and Accountability Act (HIPAA) Privacy Rule in the USA (Shabani et al. 2018). Within the Privacy Rule, the Safe Harbor standard for achieving the de-identification of personal data singles out 18 distinct identifiers, the removal of which is said to make the resulting information "not individually identifiable," and thus anonymous. Differently from this, recital 26 of the GDPR states that personal data should be considered anonymous insofar as the data subject cannot be identified "by any means reasonably likely to be used [...] either by the controller or by any other person" (GDPR recital 26; see also Article 29 Working Party,18 opinion 05/2014). To ascertain whether means are reasonably likely to be used to identify the natural person, the GDPR further states that "account should be taken of all objective factors, such as the costs of and the amount of time required for identification, taking into consideration the available technology at the time of the processing and technological developments" (recital 26).

As such, and in line with the overall decentralized thrust of the Regulation, the GDPR can be said to adopt a context-based criterion to determine whether personal data should be considered as irreversibly de-identified (and thus anonymous), while devolving to controllers the responsibility to address such a question (is there a "reasonable likelihood" that reidentification techniques can be effectively used to de-anonymize my given dataset?) in the context of their concrete processing activities.

Moreover, the definition of "anonymous data" advanced by the GDPR seems to create a "catch-22" situation (Shabani and Marelli 2019). On the one hand, as we have seen, the processing of anonymous data is not subjected to the safeguards entailed by the GDPR, and this represents an implicit incentive to the processing and sharing of anonymous information. On the other hand, however, *precisely* the absence of said safeguards, as well as the enhanced circulation of data, are factors that, in themselves, are bound to *increase* the likelihood of reidentification of the data subject, which, in turn, can lead to the de-anonymization of the dataset. Thus, the very approach toward anonymous data processing adopted by the GDPR can be said to set a high legal bar for achieving anonymization of data (Quinn and Quinn 2018)—especially in the context of the processing of genetic data (Shabani and Marelli 2019).

3.3 The "Right Balance" Between Innovation and Protection of Individuals' Rights and Interests?

As explicitly stated in the Regulation, the adoption of the GDPR has been underpinned by the aim to accomplish, at once, two seemingly contrasting objectives, namely, the protection of the fundamental rights and freedoms of individuals with regard to the processing of personal data (i.e., data protection), and the enhancement of the free movement of personal data within the EU, in view of the creation of a full-fledged Digital Single Market poised to foster digital innovation (i.e., data utility). For such "data protection–versus–data utility" conundrum, the implementation of a controller-based and decentralized approach to data protection, in place of rigid and detailed provisions, can be assessed ambivalently.

On the one hand, beside the introduction of novel rights for data subjects, the flexibility entailed by mechanisms such as the "compatibility test," as well as the enhanced role assigned to institutionalized ethics in defining the scope of data processing in Research & Innovation programs (on this aspect, cf. Marelli and Testa 2018), could be said to increase data subjects' protection while affording patients and/or research participants a substantive rather than mere formalistic engagement in the development and use of novel eHealth technologies.

On the other hand, however, in addition to the controllers' discretionary prerogatives, the GDPR upholds a far-reaching "research exemption" to the strict limitations otherwise imposed on the processing of sensitive data (art. 9(1)), for instance relaxing requirements for consent (recital 33) and limitations in data storage (art. 5(1)(e)). In addition, as per recital 159, the GDPR provides a remarkably broad definition of activities falling under the rubric of "scientific research," including "technological development and demonstration," "applied research," and "privately funded research." As a consequence, eHealth and mHealth companies (such as app providers, telemedical companies, AI companies, etc.), claiming to conduct "scientific research" activities with data gathered from individuals, stand to benefit directly from the regulatory leeway deriving from these combined provisions—with an arguably significant shift of the balance of interests in favor of data controllers over data subjects (Pormeister 2017; Marelli and Testa 2018).

In the final analysis, whether the GDPR will achieve the stated aim of ensuring the "right balance" between providing appropriate safeguards to individuals—thus allaying still widespread privacy and data protection concerns surrounding eHealth technologies (Powles and Hodson 2017)—and creating the conditions for a thriving Digital Single Market in domains such as health and care, is something that only its implementation in the coming months and years will be able to tell.

4 Ethical Issues in eHealth Technologies

Notwithstanding the similar data protection concerns raised, the expression "eHealth" (cf. Eysenbach 2001) connotes a vast array of different technologies (as well as their related social practices), each of which raises distinct ethical issues. In what follows, eHealth technologies will be divided into three broad families:

- Online eHealth (self-management tools)
- Monitoring techniques
- New and unconventional eHealth technologies

The respective ethical aspects will be discussed separately.

4.1 Online eHealth (Self-Management) Tools

One of the most widespread forms of eHealth is represented by consumers' demand for online health information, which remains "one of the most important subjects that internet users research online" (Fox 2011a). Besides dedicated websites, health-related information is increasingly being accessed through blogs and social media. According to Fox, the information most commonly searched for within this broad category is that referring to diseases and/or medical problems, medical treatment and/or medical procedure, or information regarding doctors or other health-care professionals (Fox 2011a). The same study has also shown that the vast majority of online eHealth consumers consists of people affected by chronic diseases, whose primary aim is not only that of broadening the information at their disposal but also finding "peers," that is, people affected by their same condition, with whom they can share their experiences and from whom they could receive advice and/or support.[1] Giving rise to distinct forms of "biosociality" (a term coined by renowned anthropologist Paul Rabinow (1996) to capture the emergence of new collectivities, social networks, and social interactions forming around shared biological—especially genetic—and medical characteristics), the so-called peer-to-peer health care (cf. Chap. 3) is rapidly expanding, in the USA and beyond (Fox 2011b).

By helping acquiring information with respect to health and health-related issues, eHealth technologies are said to provide individuals—independently of their literacy and/or economic status—with the opportunity "to become more informed and thus better prepared to discuss treatment plans with their physicians" (Czaja et al. 2013, p. 31; Taha et al. 2009). In particular, by facilitating peer-to-peer interactions and by allowing patients to get in touch with medical expert networks and/or patient associations, online eHealth technologies contribute to patients' acquaintance with health-related issues, thus promoting their improvement of medical literacy.

What has been just depicted as an emancipatory affordance of online eHealth tools may, however, give rise to a number of pitfalls. Firstly, the much too informed online individual may become a distrustful patient, unwilling to adhere to medical advices provided in conventional face-to-face settings (Czaja et al. 2013). Secondly, such individual may equally turn into a consumer of online commercialized products lacking clear medical or preventive benefits without adequate medical oversight—something that has been shown to occur, for instance, in the case of unproven stem cell therapies as well as Direct-to-Consumer genetic tests (cf., e.g., Wallace 2011).

Another criticality ascribed to online eHealth self-management tools concerns the way in which online eHealth information is presented and its tools are designed.

[1] Other sets of people who are likely to engage in online searches for people sharing their same health concerns include "internet users who are caring for a loved one; internet users who experienced a medical crisis in the past year; and internet users who have experienced a significant change in their physical health, such as weight loss or gain, pregnancy, or quitting smoking" (Fox, 2011b).

Indeed, despite its promise of improving access to health information, "to date many Internet-based health applications have been designed without consideration for needs, capabilities, and preferences of user group[s]" (Czaja et al. 2013, p. 31). Although it should be recalled that the group of users looking for health information online is rather heterogeneous—spanning from adults to older adults, affected by chronic as well as nonchronic conditions—these tools and platforms are often devised without considering the potential difficulties that users may encounter in navigating this information and understanding its content.

To summarize, two main sets of criticalities may be ascribed to eHealth online technologies: while the former—distrust toward medical experts, patients-turned-consumers without adequate medical oversight—represents a potential negative impact of the aforementioned technologies on online consumers, the latter—inadequacy of eHealth online tools with respect to target users—questions the appropriateness of technologies themselves to comply with the expectations set forth by their deployment.

A fruitful strategy for partially overcoming such issues may be found in the notion of *patient engagement* (cf. Chap. 1), defined as the act of involving patients—as well as the latter's availability of being involved—in their health and care processes (Gruman et al. 2010; Hibbard and Mahoney 2010; Clancy 2011; Barello et al. 2012; Menichetti et al. 2016). In broad terms, engaging patients has been considered as a key priority for contemporary health care and a policy objective in many countries (Thompson 2007). Besides fostering patients' capacity to significantly impact on the orientation, management, and evaluation of research programs concerning their diseases, "patient activation" has been associated with better adherence to treatments and improved treatment outcomes (Greene and Hibbard 2012; Vahdat et al. 2014).

In the context of the eHealth technologies under investigation here, patient engagement may lead to the design of technologies that more closely match users' preferences. Indeed, patients have been shown to adopt new technologies "if the tools are felt to be relevant to their own health-care problems, are engaging and easy to use, and are effective at achieving behaviour change" (Birnbaum et al. 2015, p. 754). As such, "without considering the patient as an active agent in the health-care environment," eHealth solutions run the risk "to be substantially ineffective in the end" (Triberti and Barello 2016, p. 151). As a consequence, "user-centered design" has been advanced as the "gold standard" for developing the eHealth tools of the future (cf. Chap. 9).

In addition, an engaged role from the part of the patients from the very onset of technological development can also reduce the risk that perceived harm related to technology usage (e.g., uncertainty about privacy rights, or about the management of one's own health data) would negatively influence users' acceptance at a later time. Indeed, despite the initial enthusiasm for eHealth technologies, some evidence exists that patients remain skeptical toward technological tools if these do not evolve in line with their changes, renewed attitudes, and needs (Currie et al. 2015; Gaul and Ziefle 2009).[2]

4.2 Monitoring Techniques

A second family of eHealth technologies is the so-called monitoring techniques, that is, the set of techniques allowing a continuous observation of one's own condition (physiological and physical) performed through body and/or home sensors. Monitoring techniques were originally developed for improving health care locally, in those contexts in which geographical distances would have precluded regular health measures. Additionally, they have been typically devised for monitoring the behavior of chronic patients and/or the elderly, while communicating relevant health and/or behavioral information in real time to health-care professionals and/or their reference family member. Amongst the broad set of monitoring techniques, an important difference exists between more conventional monitoring techniques, such as telemedicine, and rather new and unconventional monitoring techniques, such as those labeled under the rubric of "Ambient Intelligence." These two sets of monitoring systems differ profoundly not only in terms of their technological capacities and impact on patients' health, but also in terms of ethical threats potentially related to their (ab)use.

Telemedicine, which literally means "healing at a distance" (Strehle and Shabde 2006), has been defined by the World Health Organization (WHO) as "the delivery of health-care services, where distance is a critical factor, by all health-care professionals using information and communication technologies for the exchange of valid information for diagnosis, treatment and prevention of disease and injuries, research and evaluation, and for the continuing education of health care providers, all in the interests of advancing the health of individuals and their communities" (WHO 1998). According to this definition, telemedicine comprises sets of techniques aimed at overcoming the obstacles that may arise in providing assistance and/or care to a patient, using advanced telecommunication devices able to transmit medical information from the patient herself to the healthcare facility and vice versa, thus actively contributing to the improvement of health-care services. Despite their differences, the WHO has suggested to include, under the label "telemedicine," all those interventions (i) whose aim is to provide clinical support; (ii) which are intended to overcome geographical barriers, connecting users who are not in the same physical location; (iii) which involve the use of various types of information and communication technologies; (iv) whose broad goal is to improve health

[2]Actually, it is noteworthy to point out that the patient who let herself be engaged is neither a representative nor an average patient, but she is clearly a more active individual, with a better access to health care. Social determinants of health such as income, housing, social environments, and education have a real impact not only on health outcomes, but also on the opportunity to become a fully engaged patient.

outcomes (Ryu 2012, p. 9). Telemedicine applications are further classified in "store-and-forward" (or "asynchronous") interventions, in those instances in which telemedicine involves the exchange of prerecorded data between two or more individuals at different times, and "real time" (or "synchronous") interventions, when the involved individuals are simultaneously present for immediate exchange of information, as in the case of videoconferencing. Moreover, the interaction between the individuals involved may occur in the form of exchange between health-care professional and patient ("health professional-to-patient"), or between two or more health-care professionals ("health professional-to-health professional") (Ryu 2012, p. 10).

Traditional eHealth monitoring systems such as telemedicine in its different instantiations present several sets of advantages, among which the following are also ethically relevant. *Firstly* (cf. Chap. 4), they may improve health outcomes and allow patients to be assisted and/or cured in their home environments, while also reducing costs and inconveniences for patients due to prolonged admissions and hospital-based commuting. *Additionally*, they may enable the provision of high-quality home services, while prolonging as much as possible patients' independence—thus positively impacting on patients' quality of life. *Thirdly*, eHealth monitoring systems hold potential for improving health-care professionals' daily activities. Indeed, telemedicine is able to make available to the attending physician all the existing information related to the single patient and to send it, for consulting purposes, to specialists from all over the world; moreover, it contributes to reduce unnecessary administrative work, while at the same time enabling a more secure and organized management of information. *Finally*, by reducing prolonged and/or unnecessary hospitalizations, eHealth monitoring systems can also increase the efficiency and productivity of health services (Bauer 2001; Stanberry 2006). Monitoring technologies can therefore enable progress in the management and care of the chronic patient as well as of the elderly—leading to the identification of potential health problems before they become serious (cf. Chap. 5).

However, despite providing high data quality that may help ensure correct processing and interpretation of information, as well as the appropriate intervention of medical services, serious ethical concerns exist with respect to potential misuse of patients' information. In particular, the use of these technologies is usually accompanied with concerns related to *informational privacy*, that is, regarding what type of information is recorded, how it is recorded, and with whom it is shared. This appears particularly controversial in case of new and unconventional aforementioned monitoring systems, such as Ambient Intelligence.

Ambient Intelligence refers to the sets of different physical environments—such as homes, offices, meeting rooms, schools, hospitals, control centers, vehicles, tourist attractions, stores, and sports facilities (Ramos et al. 2008)—that "intelligently and unobtrusively" interact with people, through a "world of ubiquitous computing devices" (Ramos et al. 2008, p. 15), such as micro-computers and different types of sensors, in order to systematically monitor the daily activities of the target users. Despite referring to different kinds of environments, Ambient Intelligence has been bound, in recent literature (Ramos et al. 2008; Cook et al. 2009; Acampora et al.

2013), to the presence of some distinctive features: "it is context aware (it makes use of information drawn on the here-and-now situation); personalized (it is tailored on the individual user's needs); anticipatory (it develops the capacity of predicting user's needs); adaptive (it is able to modify its own functions/behavior on the basis of the user's habits); ubiquitous (it is embedded and distributed among the environment); transparent (it is able to function without direct action, nor perception, nor knowledge by the human user)" (Triberti and Barello 2016, p. 151).

As embedded in environments structurally and inherently devised to monitor human behavior, Ambient Intelligence raises at least three kinds of ethical concerns with respect to the target user that need to be considered and properly handled.

Firstly, and as already mentioned, the most relevant ethical concern regards informational privacy. In the case of Ambient Intelligence, as some scholars have noticed, almost any kind of data gathering may potentially represent a privacy violation. As an example, the use of image processing through video cameras as a potential kind of sensor has been deemed "a controversial area" (Cook et al. 2009, p. 287), as cameras filming users in specific conditions and/or while performing certain activities may appear as a violation of the individual personal sphere. In line with this observation, it is interesting to notice that, according to empirical evidence collected (Beach et al. 2009, 2010), requests for greater confidentiality exist with respect to information acquired in certain specific house areas (such as the bathroom and bedroom) where privacy violation is intuitively perceived as more serious by the side of the target user. Besides implementation of the GDPR's accountability-based approach described in the first part of this chapter, solutions exist in order to limit privacy concerns, such as limiting cameras registration to specific environments and in space obscuring bodies, but, as it has been pointed out, even seemingly innocuous ones such as walking patterns and eating habits can be combined to provide very detailed information on a person's identify and lifestyle (Bohn et al. 2005).

Secondly, and relatedly, the so-called big brother syndrome (Dwight and Feigelson 2000), that is, the negative feeling of being observed by the technology itself, may have an impact on personal behavior, inasmuch as individuals may modify their behaviors precisely as a consequence of knowing of being registered, thus limiting *de facto* their personal liberties. Ambient Intelligence technologies, in this respect, may shape individual behaviors, leading to the self-disciplining of the individual.

Finally, concerns related to the actual validity of users' authorization toward these techniques have been raised. Indeed, despite the rhetoric of transparency with respect to Ambient Intelligence systems, several doubts exist with respect to the validity of target users' consent, as the latter may be based on user's misconceptions and/or partial misrepresentation of the system and its functioning, based upon preliminary explanations that may hardly convene adequate representations of the system in which the user will be embedded. In addition to enriching the oral explanation of Ambient Intelligence systems with videos and figurative representations, a possible solution may be that of envisaging a "multistep consent" to be provided at different time points, not only before, but also in between distinct set up phases of the system.

4.3 New and Unconventional eHealth Technologies

In addition to the aforementioned and more conventional eHealth technologies, a set of novel and less conventional eHealth technologies has recently emerged and/or developed in the health and medical domains, raising distinct sets of ethical issues.

Artificial Intelligence. A first domain in which eHealth technologies are rapidly evolving revolves around the adoption of Artificial Intelligence (AI) within the medical context and, in particular, as a clinical care tool. Inasmuch as some areas of medicine, such as radiology, pathology, and dermatology, find themselves dealing with increasing amount of data, they are likely to adopt AI tools, in order to "extract fine information about issues invisible to the human eye and process those data quickly and accurately" (Jha and Topol 2016). In this context, such emerging technology may run the risk of impacting on the epistemic and social authority of physicians and medical specialists. At the same time, however, the idea that the AI will inevitably displace medical expertise and reconfigure entrenched epistemic and social relations between doctors and patients seems largely far-fetched. As analysts have noted, "given that artificial intelligence has a 50-year history of promising to revolutionize medicine and failing to do so, it is important to avoid overinterpreting these new results" (Beam and Kohane 2016, p. E2).

Virtual Reality. Virtual reality (or environment) is defined as a "spatial (usually 3D) world seen from a first person's point of view" where the view "is under the real-time control of the user" (Lányi 2006, 87). In recent years, virtual reality has rapidly emerged as a promising technology in the health-care domain, in particular in diverse sensitive settings such as aged care, clinical rehabilitation, and mental health (Valmaggia et al. 2016; Moyle et al. 2017). With regard to this latter domain, some scholars have recently observed that, because of its power to simulate the environmental conditions that trigger problems, it may be used to treat phobias, posttraumatic stress disorders, and to induce empathy and other altruistic-based behaviors in patients (Freeman et al. 2017). Moreover, inasmuch as it is an immersive technology, virtual reality has the potential to be introduced effectively in pain management, distracting chronic patients from their experience of pain (Gromala et al. 2015). In addition to some practical challenges in implementing virtual reality technologies, for example, the costs of implementation and the need for one-on-one assistance from care staff (Waycott et al. 2018), some ethical challenges may also arise. First, due to the novelty of the technology itself, possible system failures may happen, which may be interpreted by vulnerable participants as signs of failure on their part (Waycott et al. 2018, p. 412). Secondly, and more importantly, inasmuch as virtual reality involves being immersed in an alternate reality, it may amplify people's experience, creating experiences of confusions and even trauma, which may be particularly problematic for those vulnerable categories of individuals for which these techniques are deployed (Vines et al. 2017).

Virtual Worlds. A further development of virtual reality is represented by virtual worlds, consisting of technologies devised so as to provide users with the possibility to share the experience of an interactive virtual environment through the creation, customization, and use of avatars (Morie and Chance 2011), thus combining the advantages of virtual realities environments with the connectivity offered by social networks. Despite their potential impressive impact in health care, particularly as tools promoting a high level of education for health-care professionals, some doubts have been raised with respect to the involvement of patients in these settings. Indeed, inasmuch as the virtual worlds are contexts where different individuals are simultaneously present, it is not always possible to predict the (ab)use and the impact these systems will have on patients themselves (Triberti and Chirico 2017).

5 Conclusions

This contribution has explored the regulatory landscape that, after the entry into effect of the GDPR, underpins the unfolding of eHealth research and innovation in the EU. As we have observed in the chapter, the GDPR promotes a decentralized approach to data protection—centered on the accountability of data controllers. Whether this approach will be effective in achieving an effective balance between protection of the rights and interests of individuals (data subjects) and the promotion of innovation in the eHealth sector is, at the time of writing, still a major open question.

Moreover, this contribution has provided an overview of the societal and ethical challenges raised by the development of novel digital technologies, examining some important ethical issues that may arise when developing and implementing eHealth solutions for health management in the context of medical (e.g., chronic) conditions. In conclusion, we stress that, regarding the psycho-cognitive factors in P5 eHealth technologies, it is still paramount to develop a set of psychometric instruments able to capture the important psychological characteristics that would allow (1) the user (patient)-centered design of devices and interfaces, in order to tailor eHealth solutions on users' needs, and (2) the adequate technology-mediated analysis of patients' characteristics to be considered within the field of chronic illness management.

Acknowledgment This work was supported by the Project INNOVAcaRE (Enhancing Social Innovation in Elderly Care: Values, Practices, and Policies) funded by Fondazione Cariplo (V.S.) and the European Union's Horizon 2020 research and innovation program under the Marie Sklodowska-Curie grant agreement No 753531 (L.M.).

References

Acampora, G., Cook, D. J., Rashidi, P., & Vasilakos, A. V. (2013). A survey on ambient intelligence in healthcare. *Proceedings of the IEEE, 101*(12), 2470–2494.

Albrecht, J. (2016). *Conclusion of the EU data protection reform*. Available at: https://www.janalbrecht.eu/2016/04/2016-04-13-conclusion-of-the-eu-data-protection-reform/

Barello, S., Graffigna, G., & Vegni, E. (2012). Patient engagement as an emerging challenge for healthcare services: mapping the literature. *Nursing Research and Practice, 2012*.

Bauer, K. A. (2001). Home-based telemedicine: A survey of ethical issues. *Cambridge Quarterly of Healthcare Ethics, 10*(2), 137–146.

Beach, S., Schulz, R., Downs, J., Matthews, J., Seelman, K., Barron, B., & Mecca, L. (2009, October). End-user perspectives on privacy and other trade-offs in acceptance of quality of life Technology. In *Gerontologist* (Vol. 49, pp. 164–164).

Beach, S., Schulz, R., Downs, J., Matthews, J., Seelman, K., Person Mecca, L., & Courtney, K. (2010). Monitoring and privacy issues in quality of life technology applications. *Gerontechnology, 9*(2), 78–79.

Beam, A. L., & Kohane, I. S. (2016). Translating artificial intelligence into clinical care. *Jama, 316*(22), 2368–2369.

Birnbaum, F., Lewis, D., Rosen, R. K., & Ranney, M. L. (2015). Patient engagement and the design of digital health. *Academic Emergency Medicine, 22*(6), 754–756.

Bohn, J., Coroamă, V., Langheinrich, M., Mattern, F., & Rohs, M. (2005). Social, economic, and ethical implications of ambient intelligence and ubiquitous computing. In *Ambient intelligence* (pp. 5-29). Springer, Berlin, Heidelberg.

Clancy, C. M. (2011). Patient engagement in health care. *Health Services Research, 46*(2), 389–393.

Cook, D. J., Augusto, J. C., & Jakkula, V. R. (2009). Ambient intelligence: Technologies, applications, and opportunities. *Pervasive and Mobile Computing, 5*(4), 277–298.

Currie, M., Philip, L. J., & Roberts, A. (2015). Attitudes towards the use and acceptance of eHealth technologies: A case study of older adults living with chronic pain and implications for rural healthcare. *BMC Health Services Research, 15*(1), 162.

Czaja, S., Beach, S., Charness, N., & Schulz, R. (2013). Older adults and the adoption of healthcare technology: Opportunities and challenges. In *Technologies for active aging* (pp. 27-46), Boston, MA: Springer.

Dwight, S. A., & Feigelson, M. E. (2000). A quantitative review of the effect of computerized testing on the measurement of social desirability. *Educational and Psychological Measurement, 60*(3), 340–360.

EC. (2018). Communication from the Commission to the European Parliament, the European Council, the Council, the European Economic and Social Committee and the Committee of the Regions on enabling the digital transformation of health and care in the Digital Single Market; empowering citizens and building a healthier society, COM(2018)33.

Eysenbach, G. (2001). Journal of Medical Internet Research is now indexed in Medline. *Journal of Medical Internet Research, 3*(3), e25.

Fox, S. (2011a). Health topics. Pew internet and American life project February 1, 2011.

Fox, S. (2011b). *Peer-to-peer healthcare*. Pew Internet & American Life Project.

Freeman, D., Reeve, S., Robinson, A., Ehlers, A., Clark, D., Spanlang, B., & Slater, M. (2017). Virtual reality in the assessment, understanding, and treatment of mental health disorders. *Psychological Medicine, 47*(14), 2393–2400.

Gaul, S., & Ziefle, M. (2009, November). Smart home technologies: Insights into generation-specific acceptance motives. In *Symposium of the Austrian HCI and Usability Engineering Group* (pp. 312–332). Springer, Berlin, Heidelberg.

Greene, J., & Hibbard, J. H. (2012). Why does patient activation matter? An examination of the relationships between patient activation and health-related outcomes. *Journal of General Internal Medicine, 27*(5), 520–526.

Gromala, D., Tong, X., Choo, A., Karamnejad, M., & Shaw, C. D. (2015, April). The virtual meditative walk: virtual reality therapy for chronic pain management. In *Proceedings of the 33rd Annual ACM Conference on Human Factors in Computing Systems* (pp. 521-524). ACM.

Gruman, J., Rovner, M. H., French, M. E., Jeffress, D., Sofaer, S., Shaller, D., & Prager, D. J. (2010). From patient education to patient engagement: implications for the field of patient education. *Patient Education and Counseling, 78*(3), 350–356.

Hibbard, J. H., & Mahoney, E. (2010). Toward a theory of patient and consumer activation. *Patient Education and Counseling, 78*(3), 377–381.

Jha, S., & Topol, E. J. (2016). Adapting to artificial intelligence: radiologists and pathologists as information specialists. *Jama, 316*(22), 2353–2354.

Lányi, C. S. (2006). *Virtual reality in healthcare* (In *Intelligent paradigms for assistive and preventive healthcare* (pp. 87-116)). Berlin, Heidelberg: Springer.

Mager, A. (2017). Search engine imaginary: Visions and values in the co-production of search technology and Europe. *Social Studies of Science, 47*(2), 240–262.

Marelli, L., & Testa, G. (2017). *"Having a Structuring Effect on Europe": The Innovative Medicines Initiative and the Construction of the European Health Bioeconomy* (In *Bioeconomies* (pp. 73-101)). Cham: Palgrave Macmillan.

Marelli, L., & Testa, G. (2018). Scrutinizing the EU General Data Protection Regulation. *Science, 360*(6388), 496–498.

Menichetti, J., Libreri, C., Lozza, E., & Graffigna, G. (2016). Giving patients a starring role in their own care: a bibliometric analysis of the on-going literature debate. *Health Expectations, 19*(3), 516–526.

Morie, J. F., & Chance, E. (2011). Extending the reach of health care for obesity and diabetes using virtual worlds.

Moyle, W., Jones, C., Dwan, T., & Petrovich, T. (2017). Effectiveness of a virtual reality forest on people with dementia: A mixed methods pilot study. *The Gerontologist, 58*(3), 478–487.

Pormeister, K. (2017). Genetic data and the research exemption: is the GDPR going too far?.. *International Data Privacy Law*.

Powles, J., & Hodson, H. (2017). Google DeepMind and healthcare in an age of algorithms. *Health and technology, 7*(4), 351–367.

Quinn, P., & Quinn, L. (2018). Big genetic data and its big data protection challenges. *Computer Law & Security Review, 34*(5), 1000–1018.

Ramos, C., Augusto, J. C., & Shapiro, D. (2008). Ambient intelligence—the next step for artificial intelligence. *IEEE Intelligent Systems, 23*(2), 15–18.

Regulation (EU). (2016/679). General Data Protection Regulation of the European Parliament and of the Council of 27 April 2016 on the protection of natural persons with regard to the processing of personal data and on the free movement of such data, which repeals Directive 95/46/ EC.

Ryu, S. (2012). Telemedicine: Opportunities and developments in member states: Report on the second global survey on ehealth 2009 (global observatory for ehealth series, volume 2). *Healthcare Informatics Research, 18*(2), 153–155.

Shabani, M., & Marelli, L. (2019). Re-identifiability of genomic data and the GDPR. *EMBO Reports*, e48316.

Shabani, M., Dyke, S. O., Marelli, L., & Borry, P. (2018). Variant data sharing by clinical laboratories through public databases: consent, privacy and further contact for research policies. *Genetics in Medicine, 1*.

Smith, H. (2018). *Data driven healthcare: Europe to change gear*. Available at: http://www.project-pulse.eu/data-driven-healthcare-europe-to-change-gear/

Stanberry, B. (2006). Legal and ethical aspects of telemedicine. *Journal of Telemedicine and Telecare, 12*(4), 166–175.

Strehle, E. M., & Shabde, N. (2006). One hundred years of telemedicine: does this new technology have a place in paediatrics? *Arch Disease in Childhood, 91*(12), 956–959.

Taha, J., Sharit, J., & Czaja, S. (2009). Use of and satisfaction with sources of health information among older Internet users and nonusers. *The Gerontologist, 49*(5), 663–673.

Thompson, A. G. (2007). The meaning of patient involvement and participation in health care consultations: a taxonomy. *Social Science and Medicine, 64*(6), 1297–1310.

Triberti, S., & Barello, S. (2016). The quest for engaging AmI: Patient engagement and experience design tools to promote effective assisted living. *Journal of Biomedical Informatics, 63*, 150–156.

Triberti, S., & Chirico, A. (2017). Healthy avatars, healthy people: care engagement through the shared experience of virtual worlds. In *Transformative healthcare practice through patient engagement* (pp. 247–275). IGI Global.

Vahdat, S., Hamzehgardeshi, L., Hessam, S., & Hamzehgardeshi, Z. (2014). Patient involvement in health care decision making: A review. *Iranian Red Crescent Medical Journal, 16*(1).

Valmaggia, L. R., Latif, L., Kempton, M. J., & Rus-Calafell, M. (2016). Virtual reality in the psychological treatment for mental health problems: An systematic review of recent evidence. *Psychiatry Research, 236*, 189–195.

Vines, J., McNaney, R., Holden, A., Poliakov, I., Wright, P., & Olivier, P. (2017). Our year with the glass: Expectations, letdowns and ethical dilemmas of technology trials with vulnerable people. *Interacting with Computers, 29*(1), 27–44.

Wallace, H. (2011). DTC Genetic Testing: A UK Perspective, GeneWatch Report 2011. Available at [Last accessed: 5 November 2018]: http://www.councilforresponsiblegenetics.org/genewatch/GeneWatchPage.aspx?pageId=281&archive=yes

Waycott, J., Wadley, G., Baker, S., Ferdous, H. S., Hoang, T., Gerling, K., … & Simeone, A. L. (2018, May). Manipulating Reality?: Designing and Deploying Virtual Reality in Sensitive Settings. In *Proceedings of the 19th International ACM SIGACCESS Conference on Computers and Accessibility* (pp. 411–414). ACM.

WHO. (1998). A health telematics policy in support of WHO's Health-For-All strategy for global health development: Report of the WHO group consultation on health telematics, 11–16 December, Geneva, 1997. Geneva, World Health Organization.

The manufacturer's authorised representative in the EU is Springer Nature Customer Service Centre GmbH, Europaplatz 3, 69115 Heidelberg, Germany. If you have any concerns regarding our products, please contact ProductSafety@springernature.com

Printed and bound by CPI Group (UK) Ltd, Croydon, CR0 4YY
05/10/2026
02228131-0003